LIVING

POSTHUMOUSLY

LIVING
POSTHUMOUSLY

Confronting the Loss of Vital Powers

Andrew Bard Schmookler

Henry Holt and Company
New York

Henry Holt and Company, Inc.
Publishers since 1866
115 West 18th Street
New York, New York 10011

Henry Holt® is a registered
trademark of Henry Holt and Company, Inc.

Library of Congress Cataloging-in-Publication Data
Schmookler, Andrew Bard.
Living posthumously: confronting the loss of
vital powers / Andrew Bard Schmookler.—1st ed.
p.   cm.
Includes index.
1. Sickness—Psychology.   2. Loss (Psychology)   3. Life
change events.   4. Adjustment (Psychology)
5. Aging—Psychological aspects.   6. Death—Psychological
aspects.   7. Resilience (Personality trait)
8. Helplessness (Psychology)   I. Title.
R726.5.S33   1997   96-15073
616'.001'9—dc20   CIP

ISBN 0-8050-3857-4

Henry Holt books are available for special promotions
and premiums. For details contact: Director, Special Markets.

First Edition—1997

Designed by Betty Lew

Printed in the United States of America
All first editions are printed on acid-free paper. ∞

1   3   5   7   9   10   8   6   4   2

I dedicate this book to my mother

Pauline K. Schmookler

who taught me that it is not the part you're cast

to play but what you do with it.

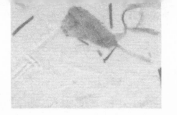

Contents

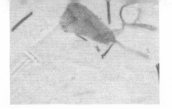

ACKNOWLEDGMENTS

One of the good things about writing a book like this is that the acknowledgments page is almost superfluous. That's because many of the benefactions for which I am most deeply grateful are already acknowledged in the text of the book itself. I am thinking of the family and friends who helped me in my confrontation with dark and difficult times. I'm thinking, too, of the health practitioners who lent their wisdom and their services to my effort to get well. To all those mentioned in the stories contained in this text, and especially to those whose roles somehow were not included in my narrative, my thanks.

For the writing of the book itself, a group of specially valued people consented to read the draft of the work and to give me their comments and encouragement. Among these are Roz Driscoll, Pauline Schmookler, Ed Schmookler, April Moore, Sara Jane Wilson, and Margee Fabyanske. If there's anyone I've forgotten, please forgive me.

For bringing the book from the draft through the successful

publication, I owe an especial debt of gratitude to my agent, Jane Dystel, who showed diplomatic skills of the highest order. To my editor, Allen Peacock, I am grateful for his role in helping me to enrich the work. And to David Groff—who for one intense week came into our lives as a professional editor and who left as a good friend—my thanks for his midwifery in helping me deliver some of the stories from the heart of my life.

And for delivering me out of the valley of the shadow, however temporarily, I give thanks to I wish I knew what.

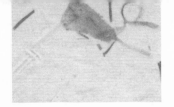

Here Today, Gaunt Tomorrow:

An Introduction

"To tell you the truth," Betty said, "you don't look so good." My wife, April, and I were visiting the Mayerses at their place in New Hampshire. Betty Mayers had not seen me in several years.

I had asked Betty for an honest appraisal, and she had given it. As I lay in bed that night, awake while everyone else in the house slept, her words haunted me.

"When I first saw you this afternoon," she had told me, "there was something scary. Like those pictures of concentration camp survivors."

Betty Mayers had known me for more than twenty years. But what she saw, she said, wasn't just the usual effects of time's passage. In part, she was responding to my involuntary disappearing act. Over the past half-year, I had—inexplicably—lost twenty pounds, and there had not been any surplus about me to begin with.

One of my favorite Woody Allen lines had been popping up in my thoughts for a while. In *Manhattan,* the character played by Woody Allen is standing next to one of those human skeletons assembled for classroom purposes. Woody is talking about what he wants his life to amount to after it's all over. Trying to find an acceptable phrase to refer to the time after his death, Woody begins the phrase "when I" and then, gesturing toward the skeleton, he continues, "thin out."

Now, as I saw myself thinning out, as my recurrent and apparently inexplicable malady was paring away my flesh, the line had become for me a bit less hilarious.

But Betty said it was not just my losing weight. The brightness in my eyes was dimming. Something about me looked not well.

I had felt "not well" for some eight years at that point, and had hardly been hesitant to admit it. Off and on—good weeks and bad weeks, good days and bad days, good hours and bad hours—I had felt my vitality sapped, and even my best times felt vaguely convalescent. I had taken this mysterious malady sufficiently seriously to pursue diagnosis and cure with relentless determination. But that night, Betty's words brought me to a new level of seriousness in my confrontation with the ongoing draining of my vital powers.

I have always expected high performance from myself, and I am by nature a problem solver, so any impediment to my well-being that arises I tend to regard with some seriousness. But at some level, regarding this unexplained debilitation, I always told myself, "This can't be anything much." There must be some little adjustment I can make—in my diet, in my body alignment, in my environment—and then everything will be fine. Underneath this annoying layer of toxicity, I thought, I am still strong and young and healthy.

The mirror of other people's eyes helped keep my worry from going too deep. They saw that I was still productive in my work—it not being visible to them that I moved through it as though weighted down, rather than alighting and leaping with a dancer's grace. I still played competitive basketball in the county league, one of the few players over forty, and still known more for my hustle than for any other asset as a player. Though I felt but a shadow of my former self, others saw me as fully embodied, still present and accounted for.

Sometimes I would fearfully remind myself that "looking good" is not always a reliable index, recalling how great my father looked at my college graduation in June 1967. By the third of October, his Hodgkin's disease had killed him. But for the most part, others' perceptions strengthened a voice in me that assured me that my problem, whatever it was, was not too big a deal.

Besides seeming okay, the great majority of the time *I did not feel terrible*. I would describe my baseline level of malaise as somewhere close to that one suffers from a moderately bad cold. Certainly not as bad as full-blown influenza. Nothing like what some kinds of cancer can do. A moderately bad cold—no big deal—not if it's gone in a week or two. You can wait to feel better, to regain your capacity for joy. But when *years* go by, distress at the level of a moderately bad cold can become burdensome, particularly when the source of that distress remains a mystery. So, on one level I worried about what was happening to me. At the same time I remained confident that beneath some vexing problem, I remained a very healthy man.

The mirror that Betty held up to me shattered that underlying feeling of confidence. My mother, too, had been expressing concern for a few months. "You're looking so gaunt," she would say. "You should eat more." After years of being concerned because I was concerned, suddenly Mom herself was really worried. But this did not really affect my own depth of apprehension. Rather I noted with amusement that, by thinning me out so noticeably, my ongoing malady was finally speaking in a language my Jewish mother could understand.

But Betty was not my Jewish mother. She was my Protestant peer. And her external confirmation of my internal sense that something scary was happening to me precipitated a deeper recognition that I was losing ground. I had taken on the restoration of my health as a veritable part-time job, consulting practitioners both conventional and un. I had explored the possibility that it was a low-grade virus, that it was chronic fatigue syndrome, that it was a matter of spinal adjustment, that it was an environmental illness. No diagnosis seemed to fit; none of the treatments got to the heart of the matter. The mystery remained unsolved, and despite my resourcefulness in devising strategies to get at the root of my difficulties and despite my conscientiousness in following the advice I could get, I was losing ground.

This was a twin blow—being forced to confront both the possibility of defeat despite my best efforts, and the prospect of never again enjoying my vital powers. It was after absorbing this blow that I decided to write this book.

I realized that both those experiences that I was finding so bitter and frightening were an inevitable part of human life. Ultimately, for all of us, our efforts to maintain our vitality will fail, our most treasured capabilities will slip out of our grasp. Even if I should find that magic bullet I had sought so long and dispel the hated cloud hovering over me, it would be a mere stay of execution. Eventually I—as well as everyone else—would lose my vital powers. If not through the sort of chronic illness that had somehow unaccountably gained a choke hold on my life, then through the inescapable process of aging and, finally, death.

As obvious as this may be, it still came to me as an important if unwelcome realization. And I felt the time had come to change my posture toward this experience.

After years of fighting against what had seemed so unacceptable a loss, I found myself pondering the possibility that perhaps there was something to be gained from accepting it, from acknowledging to myself: "This is my experience and I might as well see what I can learn from it." Rather than ceaselessly chafing against all the ways my disability impeded my creative expression, I wondered if I might do better to see what I could create out of it. After all, if the loss of vital powers—which I was rejecting as a personal affront—is an inescapable part of the human condition, perhaps what I could learn from embracing my experience others might find worthwhile learning with me.

In this way, my ongoing distress could be transformed into grist for my mill. In this, I see, I will be repeating an important pattern in my previous work. All my previous books have grown out of pain: the pain of seeing how out of joint is the civilization in which we live, how tormented and destructive, how out of balance it is with the living energies of this beautiful planet. I have consistently channeled the acute distress I have felt at witnessing this global dysfunction into creative work devoted first to understanding and then to helping correct the harmful forces at work. Each item of news that would otherwise hurt me to see is thus transmuted into matter for my endeavor.

As much as it has pained me to see the wounds of the earth, the present pain was rather closer to home. It is one thing to be a healthy animal running in distress in the midst of a diseased world. When the disease is within one's very flesh, the pain of recognition has a different quality. And embarking upon the spiritual and intellectual exploration of this experiential space seemed fraught with greater uncertainty.

If I continue to be debilitated, I wondered, will I have the strength to illuminate the challenge I face in confronting my decline? If my dullness of spirit persists, will I possess the sensitivity and intensity to plumb the meaning of my loss? Embarking on my project, the very instrument by which I would investigate the pain of limitation and disability was itself limited and disabled.

On the other hand, if—God willing—my health should be restored during the unfolding of this project, I also wondered, will I maintain the interest to see it through to completion? For so long, I had yearned for a return to what I have taken to be my true self—highly energetic, resilient, ready to take on the world. Would I not be tempted to turn away from the realm of weakness and finitude as soon as my moment-to-moment experience would allow it?

Only time would tell which of these dilemmas I would face, and whether the project would survive my resolution of it. I knew only that my attention was being pulled toward this world of illness and suffering, with its portents of the inescapability of ultimate decline and death. It was now time to regard my affliction not just as an annoyance and distraction, but also as an opportunity.

There is a genre of nonfiction literature in which a sick person recounts the story of his or her illness, providing an autobiographical travelogue of the land of disease. This book will not be of that genre. I have appreciated reading many of these works, often feeling at the conclusion of the book a sense of intimacy and even friendship with the author who has shared his or her (usually her) experience. But spinning such a narrative is not the way my mind works.

My own story concerns me here less for the sake of its own drama than as a means of exploring some larger questions about the human condition that my experience has raised in my mind. I am happy to share myself in the course of this exploration, and indeed I believe that in pursuing such human matters, a degree of personal openness is an indispensable element of meaningful communication. And so my own experience will be a recurrent thread, but more for the purpose of illuminating larger questions than as an end in itself. I am regarding my illness as a passport that has taken me to a realm of human experience that countless others have entered before me and that lies ahead of all the rest of us. With this passport in hand, I am asking: How do we deal with the discovery and the experience of the transitoriness of our powers and of our very lives?

The book is divided into three parts. The first concerns loss: loss of a sense of control, loss of an old identity, loss of comforting illusions. The second concerns the possibilities for rebirth, for finding a rich and meaningful life in the new terrain on which, after such losses, one finds oneself. And the third concerns the meaning for our lives of the inescapable fact that they do not go on forever.

PART I

Losing It

CHAPTER 1

Beneath It All There Is No Bottom

How Much Do We Control What Happens to Us?

As an American male, I was taught a great deal more about how to win than about how to deal with loss.

TAKING MEASURES

Even before the ball hit the rim, I had a good idea where I should position myself to get the rebound. But Big Barney was parked in the vicinity, and I knew all too well that what he lacked in finesse he made up for by throwing his weight around. Adhering to my new policy for playing basketball, I refrained from my usual move for the rebound.

My new policy could be easily summarized: no collisions. The purpose of this policy, as of several other measures I had taken over the course of the season, was to see if I could escape from my chronic postgame fate. Each week, after driving home from a night of basketball with a bunch of other middle-aged guys at a school gym in Chevy Chase, Maryland, I'd feel invigorated. I loved the feeling of being cleansed and renewed that came from sweating until my shirt was wet and breathing deep until my ribs moved smoothly. But always two hours after the game was over, the sick feeling would descend on me: a terrible headache, a hangover that would last until well into the following day. Along with the pain came an enervation that was more than a mirror image of the invigoration of the night before.

I'd guessed earlier that it might have something to do with overheating. Probably all the other guys, when they got into their cars after the game, were also steaming up all the windows. But I sensed that maybe all that internal combustion wasn't working for me. When I tuned in to how my head felt while I was playing, I thought: "Too hot. My brains are boiling. It's throwing me off." So I had rigged up a wet headband to act as a cooling system. My sense of overheating diminished, but the headaches persisted. Two hours. I could almost set my clock by it.

Perhaps the problem was that my spine was being compressed too much. Even my more sedentary daily life seemed to require me to lapse occasionally into yoga postures like the plow; I would stretch the muscles of my upper back and neck to keep myself from being strung too tight, like a bow drawn to shoot arrows off behind me. Importing this remedy into my weekly basketball game, I began the practice of doing the postures during breaks in the games. Yoga is great stuff, but it didn't prevent my postgame hangover.

Neither did the various other remedies that had been recommended by an M.D. (take magnesium supplements) or by a practitioner of alternative medicine (soak your wrists and ankles in a tub of cold water after the game). So now I was trying a new policy: avoid collisions.

My game had always been physical, perhaps foolishly so for someone a couple inches under six feet, and more than a little under 160 pounds. But I decided that perhaps the problem was that my head—setting, as some body workers had noted, not too firmly on the column of my neck—could no longer take the pounding and jostling inflicted by my customary style of play. In order to continue my basketball career, and preserve myself from my weekly agony, I had made a compromise: keep playing, but be more discreet in courting impact. Dart in, dart out. It felt a bit sissified, this "float like a butterfly, sting like a bee" style of play. But if it worked . . .

The policy worked—in the sense that I managed to get through the whole evening without bumping into anyone. My head was neither overheated nor askew on my neck. But two hours later, my nasty friend the hangover was making himself at home. Sitting on the edge of the tub with my wrists and ankles dangling into the cool water, I grasped that whether I won or lost at basketball, my malady was continuing to defeat me.

Although I loved basketball, not only for the pleasures of the game itself but also because the jousts on the court renewed my sense of my young manhood, that game was not what my life was about. But basketball was not the only theater of this war.

From basketball I could always retreat. But eating is a necessary engagement. Facing the choice between "Eat and feel sick" and "Don't eat," I felt my war against my sickness inescapably thrust upon me.

And, of course, I was determined to win it.

THERE'S GOTTA BE A REASON

Post hoc ergo propter hoc (Latin for "after this, therefore because of this") is a logical fallacy, one of the ways a thinker is taught not to think. But sometimes, I've discovered, it's the best a person can do.

I did not feel sick every time I ate. Eating wasn't like putting a gun to my head and shooting myself. It was more like Russian roulette. Often the chamber was empty, and after I ate, life would just go on as it always had. But not seldom, after I ate, the cloud of malaise would descend. My whole system would feel somehow polluted, befogged. But what determined whether I would get away with eating or be struck down by it? I had to find out.

It was this need to know, combined with my malady's cleverness in encrypting its secrets, that gave me a better understanding of how superstitious thinking arises in the human comedy.

I had always regarded superstitious people with some condescension, dismissing their way of thinking as childish and irrational. Like some baseball player who for every game must wear his "lucky socks," the ones he was wearing when he hit the home run in the World Series: *post hoc,* he figures, *ergo.* . . . But now, my experience with food brought me to see that superstitious thought can represent a person's best effort to find an explanation when confronted with a question both mysterious and vital.

If a problem is important enough, "I haven't got a clue" is really less satisfactory than some hypothesis, however tenuous. If the answer to some urgent question is sufficiently obscure, *post hoc* is not so much a fallacy as the best available means of generating a hypothesis.

For me, the arena for this kind of thinking was my ingestion of food. It had long been clear that eating was somehow a trigger of my symptoms: "after eating therefore because of eating" becomes persuasive after a sufficient number of instances. But why some times and not others? What is the relevant factor? Fact is, I didn't have much of a clue. But it was too important a question to accept being wholly clueless. I was reduced to thinking, "I feel lousy and we had eggplant tonight. I remember I felt bad after an eggplant meal last year, too." Post hoc, and voila, not eating eggplant became my version of wearing my lucky socks.

But just like the baseball player who doesn't keep hitting home runs just because he wears the socks, I wasn't managing to shake off my symptoms.

I grew determined to bring "the light of science"—controlled experiment—to dispel the mists of superstition. I decided I would now investigate the diet question with rigor to the nth degree. This newly ruthless determination was the culmination of several years of close observation and various less tightly controlled experiments to identify what foods I might be allergic or reactive to.

THE QUEST

I gave up on conventional medicine after a few attempts: my symptoms did not match any known pattern; my physicals and lab work disclosed nothing; physicians of good reputation said they could not help me. So I turned to other approaches.

For a good while, I worked with Charles Gilliam, an excellent cranial-sacral therapist, to see if his work might alleviate my chronic feeling of distress and fatigue where my neck joins my head and where it joins my upper back. My head didn't feel screwed on right, as I told Charles, and I wondered if that might be connected with a chronic feeling of tightness in the muscles of my eyes, as if I were working against taut rubber bands when I moved my eyes from side to side or up and down. Accompanying that discomfort was an intermittent lethargy which meant that, while some days I could play basketball, there were days it took a big effort to climb a flight of stairs. Worst of all was a general loss of spark at the emotional and spiritual levels. A low-hanging cloud hung over my world, leaving the mundane levels visible enough but obscuring all higher vistas.

Charles's work was excellent, and I always left his therapeutic table feeling clearer and lighter. After a time, however, I came to feel that the cranial-sacral work was merely treating the symptoms;

after each session the problem would keep leaking back into me like water into a well once the pump is turned off. Though there seemed to be a variety of contributors to this seepage—exertion, sleep problems, the quality of the suburban air I breathed—the evidence had become quite strong that something in my response to food was replenishing the well of my discomfort.

I was referred to Dr. James Johnson in Washington, D.C., who proved to be a very caring and generous doctor. J.J. (as he was called) suggested I begin by eliminating the usual food allergy suspects. I had shown a tendency to allergy in general from the moment I was born: they put the legally required silver nitrate in my eyes just in case my mother had syphilis. (The next day, as my father looked at me through the nursery window, the fellow next to him pointed at my swollen and discolored face and, not knowing he was addressing the father, said: "That one looks like he's been in a fight." To which my father replied: "Yeah, but you should have seen the other guy." I've always thought that a good deal of what might be called my karma is discernable in that scene.) So food allergy seemed a reasonable line of investigation.

For two months, I ate no wheat, corn, peanuts, dairy products, or eggs. The problem remained. J.J. suggested I try a particular test, though it was costly, that could generate from a vial of my blood a list of foods to which I am reactive. It was not, he said, 100 percent accurate, but it had helped some people. If this would be the key to resuming normal life, the cost was not so great, and so I embarked on this course of action.

The list that came back led to my avoiding, with utmost scrupulousness, a great variety of foods for more than two years. April, my wife, became adept at cooking and baking with no eggs, dairy products, or numerous other ingredients. I meanwhile touched not a drop of wine or coffee or black tea, avoided the dread rutabaga, eschewed lemon and paprika, kept away from sardines and shellfish.

Even this place—flowing with no milk—proved not to be the promised land.

At the time, taking that blood test and conforming my diet to fit the results seemed an extreme measure. I had always been an omnivore, known for my healthy appetite and diverse tastes, and never having to worry about how much I ate. A pleasure for the good cook to have at the table. Now I became a problematic dinner guest, and my interactions with waiters were considerably more elaborate than I (or they) would have chosen. But when my problems continued, and when eating still seemed a major trigger, I was determined to go to still greater lengths.

The reputation of that blood test was deteriorating—something about the vagaries of the interpretive process. So, for some time, I played a gustatory version of the game of Mastermind. That's the game in which one makes a guess about the identity of, say, a random four-digit number and gets a response like: You have one of the numbers correct, but even that is not in the place you have proposed. You then continue, systematically and with whatever deductive skill you can muster, to propose four-digit numbers, generating more information in response, until you know all four numbers and their proper order.

Since the effects of food allergy (or food intolerance) can allegedly begin any time up to a day or two after consumption, the total variety of foods a person eats in a two-day period poses a version of Mastermind considerably more complex than the quest for a particular four-digit number. If I woke up miserable in the morning, I would conclude that something I ate recently was a food I should avoid. If I felt fine, I could conclude that everything I had eaten was okay. (All this was, of course, based on the assumption—which I shared with a variety of my health practitioners—that I suffered from food allergy that somehow had developed as I got older.)

Dr. Sherry Rogers of Syracuse, New York, has a national reputation for helping people with allergy problems and environmental illness. A pilgrimage to Syracuse seemed a worthwhile undertaking, so April and I, and our two-year-old son, Nathaniel, made the trek north. We decided to make the trip, as much as possible, into a family adventure.

I learned some useful specifics from Sherry Rogers. She said that a rotation diet was the only reliable way of identifying what foods one reacted to. I decided that for at least four weeks, I would do the most strenuous and scrupulous procedure possible, distilled from plans I gathered from Dr. Rogers and from three or four books on the subject I checked out from the library.

After years of half-measures that brought me no answers, I was determined that this time I would compel nature to disclose the code to me. I was resolved that this time I would have either gained possession of the answer or established that the question was the wrong one. At the end, I was not going to wonder: what if I had done it more thoroughly?

This is what going whole-hog on the rotation diet meant: (1) I would eat only one food at a time. By a food, I don't mean something like "meat loaf." That has more than one ingredient. One food means something like a bowl of steamed peas with nothing on them, or a banana, or a grilled fish with nothing on it. (2) I would eat no more frequently than once every four hours. (3) I would eat no food more often than once every four days. (4) I would eat no two foods *from the same family* more than once every four days.

This last point meant learning about the arcane subject of food families, collections of foods that are genetically and chemically closely enough related that sensitization to one can spill over into sensitization to another. Some of these kinships are fairly straightforward: in a given four-day period, a person might have either a serving of beef *or* a serving of something made from cow's milk, either some chicken *or* eggs. Some of the family relationships were surprising: who would have thought that, in planning your meals, you would have to choose between having some kind of lettuce and having sunflower seeds?

But most of all, the requirement that one avoid an incestuous relationship among foods entering one's digestive tract was onerous. Consider that wheat, rice, corn, rye, oats, and barley are all in the family of grains, and that one serving of any of them prohibited consumption of any other member of the group for four full days. Likewise with the family of legumes: peas, lentils, kidney beans, peanuts, lima beans, and so forth. One visit only to that family in any given ninety-six-hour period. How do you get enough to eat? Mavericks like buckwheat (nothing to do with wheat, not a grain) and quinoa are few and far between. I could scavenge the supermarket for all the oddball foods—pomegranate, kiwi, and so forth—but it would still be a struggle to get enough to eat.

No matter. I was determined to get an answer to my question if it killed me. And get an answer I did, and it didn't kill me; it just exacted fifteen pounds of my flesh.

Four weeks later, I sat at my dining room table with the elaborate records spread out before me—detailing for more than thirty days what I ate when and how I felt when, like some grotesque game of Mastermind. I had run and rerun certain experiments to see what was coincidence and what was cause and effect. Only one thing became crushingly clear: though feeling bad was often the aftermath of eating (life would be simpler if I could have fasted indefinitely) there was no clear relationship between what I ate and how I felt. After five years of diverse programs of scrupulous avoidance, the puzzle remained.

As I sat there, thinned out and disheartened, Faust's words echoed in my mind:

Hier steh' ich vor dem Tor
Und weiss nicht mehr als bevor.

(Here I stand before the door
And know not more than before.)

For Faust, the scene was a prelude to his making a bargain with the devil that would end his impasse. But I found no one to offer me a bargain to break me out of mine.

MY BARGAIN WITH THE WORLD

When I decided to transform my malady from an impediment to my work to its subject matter, I visited some libraries and entered into a conversation of sorts with some of my fellow creatures who have also wrestled with the kind of physical decline with which I was grappling. This has long been a major part of my own reflective process. Sitting with my own experience is indispensable, but I tend to be an interactive thinker, best able to develop my own perspective through responding to the ideas of others. I cannot long sustain a line of thought in complete isolation. I also spoke with a number of people, but while many of us have given thought to illness and aging and death, I find that few of us carry our thoughts very many steps unless we are driven to do so by the persistence of inquiry the writing of a book requires. So, for the kind of conversation I wanted, the library was an important stop.

I made a surprising discovery right off: for the first time in more than a quarter-century of doing library research, I found that my local public libraries (of Shenandoah and Rockingham Counties in Virginia) were at least as useful to me as the big university libraries. For me, whose previous work had been largely on "big picture" issues of civilization and its problems, this helped underscore something else distinctive about my new undertaking: most people find the problem of illness and health, of vitality and mortality, of more immediate concern in their lives than such problems as war and peace and the fate of the biosphere. Not more important, necessarily, in the great scheme of things, but certainly more on the scale of our daily lives. Public libraries specialize in the "news you can use" kind of book, so I found there a wealth of works on how people deal with the slings and arrows of various misfortunes that can befall us.

As I read through the titles on the public library shelves, I was struck by something in their tone. I felt transported to some silent pep rally, complete with placards like "Winning Over This Disease," "You Can Lick That Disease," and "Visualize Yourself to Perfect Health." I didn't see a book called "Mortality Is Optional," but maybe I just didn't look hard enough.

This spirit of the triumph of one's will over any adversity is one that I know well from the inside. Coming out of my adolescence, I believed that by sheer dint of will and effort, I could overcome whatever obstacles I put my mind to. When I was fourteen, the doctors said that the damage to my mouth caused by the impact of a baseball would result in the death of five teeth and would require plastic surgery on my gums. I set my will to work. A few weeks later, the doctors changed their opinion on all counts; I, of course, ascribed it to my willpower. When I was seventeen, and was to play the Cowardly Lion in a high school play, I became determined to overcome a lisp that had beset me from the beginning of speech, one that had defied a half-dozen school speech therapists. By opening night, having ingrained into habit a new way of making an "S" sound that one of those therapists had shown me four years before, I had overcome the lisp. Yes, the spirit of overcoming was one I knew well.

That spirit, indeed, lies at the core of what I have come to recognize as a central bargain between me and the world. It was only as the agreement was violated by the other party that its terms became clear to me.

The first violation occurred during my early twenties, when I applied for a variety of jobs—mostly in teaching—that I knew I could perform. I pursued them vigorously, and I was rejected. With my hard-won Harvard *summa cum laude* in hand, I was outraged. My outrage pointed to my implicit bargain with the world: I discovered that I assumed the world would reward me according to my effort and merit. I never expected anything to come easily. I've never even particularly wanted things to come easily. I'm willing to work hard and long, bringing to bear all my capacities, to achieve my goals. I'm even willing to keep my goals reasonable. But if I work hard enough, if I do the right things, I should get a commensurate result.

So I worked hard, and felt betrayed when the world didn't honor our deal. (The discovery that the real world of bureaucratic organizations worked very differently from the terms of our presumed bargain was disillusioning, and the consequent feeling that I had been personally betrayed doubtless helped prepare me for the critical view of the workings of civilization that I later developed.)

Civilization may not honor its agreement to reward me for good work, but as I discovered subsequently, I maintained a belief that the natural order of things would abide by the terms of some unstated bargain. If I take good care of myself, I figured, I would stay healthy. I'm not one of those guys who thinks he can abuse his body in whatever ways suits his fancy and still be healthy. While hitchhiking in the early 1970s, for example, I met a man from Topanga Canyon near Los Angeles who smoked cigarettes and maintained that he would suffer no ill effects from his smoking because he didn't *believe* he would, and that his positive attitude would protect him. My bargain with the world was considerably more reasonable than that.

I've always eaten healthfully. At the beginning of my adulthood, I read Adelle Davis, and since then I've tended to live in the wheat-germ-and-yogurt lifestyle. I've generally stayed in good physical condition, with regular exercise. Getting up in the middle of the night, night after night, with my first two children played havoc with my sleep cycle for some years thereafter, but I always made sleep a priority and made time for sleep. I've had my share of stress in life, but I've done what I could to ease the burden of those stresses—meditating, yoga, getting good counsel as needed. In short, I worked at maintaining my health at the highest level I could.

Once my health began to deteriorate, my efforts to take good care of myself intensified. I worked hard, and as the years went by I enlisted the help of good people in a variety of healing arts. But after eight years of applying my will and my intelligence and my resources, I was still losing ground.

Thus the spirit of mastery in those books on the library shelves, though part of my own makeup, was not what the doctor ordered, as it were, when the futility of my efforts to win led me to undertake this book. The challenge for me at that time in my life was not how to win, but how to deal with the fact of losing if and when that fact appeared inescapable.

I had finally come to the point where I could see this new quest not as defeatist, but as a profound spiritual challenge. Solving problems was something I could do as well as anyone I knew, but when it came to living with a problem that could not be solved, I was lousy at it. The kind of acceptance that twelve-step programs have in mind when they speak of "accepting what cannot be changed" I could not find in my repertoire. It felt like being resigned to my defeat, and "resignation" was something I'd hand in before I could accept the unacceptable.

Ed Muller, a friend and mentor of mine living in Tucson, Arizona, has a son who was brain-damaged at birth, thanks to a drunken obstetrician. In the late 1970s, when I worked with Ed—a gifted bioenergetic analyst—I saw this boy regularly and heard his inarticulate autistic rage as teachers tried to educate some human sociability into his wounded being. My own beloved firstborn son was then a toddler, and I marveled that Ed could go on, could bear it, could be a wonderful and intact human being despite his only son's having been damaged before he had even begun. If such a situation had happened in my life, I imagined I would continually be trying to "solve" the problem, to make the grim reality go away. I would get "hung up" the way a computer "crashes" and all you can do is press the Reset button. But there is no Reset button on me.

Even though I'm not much of a praying man, when I would see someone forced to accept the unacceptable—like Ed Muller with his son, or a person forced to live with a colostomy bag, or someone else caring for a spouse with Alzheimer's disease—I would nonetheless pray that God would spare me such an ordeal. I would be hardworking and careful, and thus the world would keep its bargain and keep the unacceptable at bay. But once again, I discovered that in my bargain with the world, my signature was the only one on the contract.

What was happening to my vitality in the supposed prime of my life I did not find acceptable, yet I could not change it. In my pursuit of victory over my problem, my efforts were as good—as persevering, as comprehensive, as meticulous, as clever in terms of strategy—as any I have ever put forth. But they did not bring victory. If anything, my usual way of coping may have compounded my distress.

For me, therefore, the challenge was not to win, but to learn to live with defeat, to come to terms with terms I would not have chosen. The purpose of this book, then, is not to offer a path to perfect health or immortality. It is, rather, to explore the challenge that we all face in light of the fact that, despite our best efforts, we will ultimately have to relinquish all that we prize in ourselves. I have come to see that the triumph-of-the-will school of thought has both its uses and its abuses. The emphasis on how we can control our destiny sometimes brings out important truth, but sometimes also fosters some injurious illusions.

IN CONTROL

Nothing in my experience has led me to question the importance of taking good care of oneself. Despite my disappointment with my own present results, I continue to do all the things I know to do to maintain my body and spirit in the best possible condition. An impressive body of research is accumulating that indicates that many of the discomforts and disabilities we have believed to be automatic concomitants of the aging process are brought on or greatly accelerated by the cumulative effects of certain ways of living. To me, vitality is sufficiently sacred that I will eat, exercise, sleep, work, and conduct my life generally in ways that will preserve as much of my life energies for as long as possible.

But it is important to recognize that we are dealing here only in probabilities. It is like driving carefully. It is no guarantee that some drunk truck driver won't come crashing across the median and slam into you (as happened to the wife of a colleague of mine). Likewise, "right living" is no talisman against the health equivalent of such a car wreck.

In her book *Last Wish,* about her mother's agonizing cancer, Betty Rollin tells how the disease violated her mother's implicit belief "that she was in control and if she did the right thing (i.e., ate the right thing) everything would come out right and she would be healthy."[1] How could she have cancer when her eating habits were "unimpeachable"? I recognized myself in her anguished surprise, and as I have read more such accounts, I have seen that such surprise is common among people whom the misfortune of disease befalls.

The triumph-of-the-will school also has something important to teach when it comes to living with disease. The people who write autobiographical accounts of their illnesses tend to be independent, activist, and strong-willed. They are, on the whole, an admirable lot. I respect how Suzy Szasz—who tells her story in *Living with It*—with sheer stubborn will made a life for herself despite her lifelong struggle with lupus. Likewise I appreciate how Moira Griffin, whose book *Going the Distance* is subtitled *Living a Full Life with Multiple Sclerosis and Other Debilitating Diseases,* remained a positive, bright, and engaging young woman despite having to carry the burden of the damage inflicted on her by her multiple sclerosis. I know how pain and disappointment can quench the flame, can make it tempting to roll over and quit, and I unambivalently salute those whose will to live allows them to rise up from adversity, like some natural bonsai tree sprouting up from the face of a sheer rock cliff.

I also value the contribution made by those—Norman Cousins and Bernie Siegel are two very prominent examples—who stress how the forces of health can be fortified by the power of a positive, take-charge approach to a serious chronic illness. In their emphasis on the influence of emotion and belief on the body's capacity to maintain or restore health, such medical teachers help to correct an evident defect in some of our established philosophies of health care. One of the unfortunate consequences of an overly mechanistic understanding of the world has been a tendency of modern medicine to treat the patient as if he or she were just an elaborate machine. Just as the dominant American psychology banished mind and consciousness from its picture of the human being, so has mainstream scientific medicine tended to neglect the role of the person within the body—someone whose thoughts and feelings can have a profound impact on the healing process.

In his book *The Healing Heart,* Norman Cousins tells about encountering a man who had suffered a heart attack on the golf course and was being ministered to by a team of paramedics—or rather, his vital signs were being conscientiously attended, while the man himself went unaddressed. The man was in a panic, evidence of which Cousins saw on the cardiograph monitor in the form of a potentially lethal tachycardia (rapid heartbeat). As the paramedics worked, Cousins spoke to the man. "Sir, you've got a great heart," Cousins told him. "Why do you say that?" the man asked. To which Cousins replied, as he puts it, "rounding the sharp corners of the truth": "Sir, I've been looking at your cardiograph and I can see that you're going to be all right." After this reassurance, Cousins reports, "in less than a minute, the cardiograph showed unmistakable evidence of a slowing down of the heartbeat. . . . I looked at the man's face; the color began to return."[2]

Fear can kill, and hope can give life. We've all heard how a person, hearing of a death sentence from a witch doctor of his culture, can simply die in a short time, though he had previously been in good health. That our own doctors can wield similar powers, if unwittingly, is brought home by an anecdote told by Bernie Siegel. A woman called her husband, who was hospitalized for cancer, to see how he was feeling. He said he was fine, but when she arrived fifteen minutes later, he was dead. "In the interim, Ray, who'd been in and out of the hospital several times, had asked his doctor when he'd be able to leave. After the reply, 'Oh, I don't think you'll make it this time,' he died within minutes."[3]

Nor can the power of the placebo effect be minimized. In his books on health, written in the last decade of his life, Cousins documents the power of the placebo—a presumably inert substance given to a patient who thinks it to be a medicine—to provoke profound curative physiological response. Positive thinking is no small thing in the realm of health and healing. Truly, believing is seeing.

In telling us about these powers, people like Cousins and Siegel not only help remedy defects in some mainstream medical approaches, but also help correct a corresponding passivity among the public at large. Too many of us have learned to see ourselves as powerless to maintain health or confront disease. We see disease as something that makes us helpless victims. Being cured is something that others do to us.

There is, however, a darker side to the growing cult of control. It has to do with guilt and blame, and it is rooted in illusion and wishful thinking.

THE ILLUSION OF CONTROL

We humans naturally tend to interpret suffering as a form of punishment. Whether it be the bubonic plague or the Lisbon earthquake, history shows that when a terrible blow befalls a people, the assumption is that their suffering is a consequence of their sins. Maybe it is a cultural belief system that underlies such an interpretation. But it appears that even small children are disposed to believe that the bad things that happen to them must be their fault. If the child's parents get divorced, the psychologists say, the child is likely to take the blame upon him- or herself.

Whether this is human nature—some part of how nature assembled an animal who must learn to distinguish right from wrong, using the rewards and punishments that its environment metes out in response to various ways the creature conducts itself—or whether this interpretive reflex is embedded in particular kinds of culture, it is unfortunate that insult is so often added to injury. To bear the misfortune of having a painful illness is injury enough without having also to insult yourself with the question: What did I do to deserve this?

If I were inclined to believe that I must somehow have brought my misfortune upon myself, it would seem logically to follow that I would similarly believe that the misfortunes of others must somehow be of their own doing. But when it comes to relating to the misfortunes of others, an additional and equally destructive dynamic is at work. The healthy, it seems, have a powerful motive to perceive the ill as responsible for their ills, and with this imputation of responsibility the community tends to drive a wedge between themselves and the least fortunate among them, driving them out into an emotional wilderness like the scapegoats of ancient times.

In the contemporary literature by the ill and their advocates, a lament about this tendency to "blame the victim" appears like a threnody. "Surely you did something to bring it on yourself," writes Moira Griffin, articulating the popular attitude to which chronically ill people like herself are chronically subjected.[4] Susan Sontag, in the famous work inspired by her bout with cancer, expresses her bitterness at the way patients are "instructed" that they have caused their disease, however unwittingly, and that they also deserved it.[5]

For eight years, I have struggled with whatever this problem of mine is. I have also been open with my friends about this as well as about other, happier aspects of my life. As a result, I have had considerable opportunity of my own to witness this tendency. In a friendly way, many have been quick to suppose that my somatic discomforts must be the outward and physical sign of something askew in my inward spiritual state. One friend in particular consistently tried to pin my illness onto my chest like a lack-of-merit badge. "Must be something off in your spiritual life," he tells me. "Get inner peace and this physical stuff will take care of itself. You've got to get your life in better balance." Between the lines was the assumption, "If you aren't feeling right, you're doing something wrong."

Not knowing just how to understand my difficulties, I have seriously considered this possibility. But the alacrity with which some of my healthy friends have seized upon the idea that I must be the creator and not the victim of my predicament has bothered me. The eagerness with which some *assume* to be true what they have no way of knowing also posed a puzzle: what's in it for them to precipitate what for me is a source of bewilderment into this particular certainty?

One clue was how it *felt* for me to be "helped" by such helpful counsel: it created distance where I had hoped for the closeness of comfort and sympathy. Too distant for comfort. At times, with friends like the one pushing inner peace, I felt that my pain, rather than being taken on empathically, was being shoved back at me. So why the distance? Here, I think, is the answer: the better to make it clear that "It has happened to you and not to me, and it happened to you for reasons that assure me that I can keep it from happening to me."

I'm not the only one, I've discovered, to reach this interpretation. Moira Griffin's multiple sclerosis manifests itself intermittently, allowing her to see alternately how people treat the healthy and the ill. The ill, she says, make the healthy uneasy by reminding them of their own vulnerability.[6] But the feeling of vulnerability is not tolerable to many people. It is more reassuring to believe that if I do everything right, everything will be all right for me. It is to rescue this fantasy of control that some who are healthy feel impelled to place blame on the sick. "People terrified of illness," write Paul Levitt and Elissa Guralnick in their book on coping with serious illness, "want the comforting insurance that virtue leads infallibly to health. So they're glad to be convinced that disease never strikes except when the victim's misbehaved."[7]

As in so many tragedies of the scapegoating process, fear rather than hostility is the primary motivation.

The parents of chronically ill and handicapped children, according to Howard Brody in *Stories of Sickness,* are frequently blamed by their social peers. The blaming assumption that "if only the family had done everything right, the handicap would somehow have been prevented" is necessary to buttress the defensive belief that such a disaster "could never happen to 'good people like us.' "[8] No attack intended; it is just for the purpose of defense. But as is so often the case, our defenses give offense.

I cannot assume a posture of superiority toward the people who employ these defensive maneuvers. Like Griffin, I vacillate between comparative health and sickness. My sickness, unlike hers, does not make me wobble like a drunk or otherwise render me conspicuously ill. I cannot, therefore, match her vantage point for seeing how others treat me differentially. What I can do, however, is watch the swings in *my own* attitudes, and what I see does not always delight me. When I am one of the sick, I look at the world through that prism, humbled by my affliction. (On this, see more in Part II.) But when I feel good for a few days, I observe how readily I resume entertaining such thoughts as, "I'd never get cancer, like so-and-so; look at what good care I take of myself." And I observe my pleasure from this illusion of invulnerability and superiority, from the myth that I and only I hold the steering wheel of my fate.

If I'm good, I'll be rewarded. By a kind of magical thinking, I assure myself that the domain that I can control will in turn control those other domains where fearsome threats lie.

In the growing body of thought and belief about the connection between the emotional and spiritual realms and the somatic realm, I see an admixture of intellectual progress and infantile regression. In part, this perspective represents an advance of enlightenment in recognizing the deep ways that what we think and feel and do are connected with what happens to us. But in part also it reflects a childish reversion to a world where wishes become reality.

At the time of the plague in the sixteenth and seventeenth centuries, according to historian Keith Thomas, it was widely believed that "the happy man would not get plague."[9] How different from this is Bernie Siegel's statement that "all disease is ultimately related to a lack of love"?[10]

It's evidently difficult for us to achieve a balanced view of things. Again and again, I have observed a tendency in our culture for one extreme position to give rise not to a more balanced view but to an equally unbalanced though diametrically opposite view. Knee-jerk hawks are answered by knee-jerk doves; an excessive emphasis on personal responsibility helps give rise to a wanton infatuation with assertion of individual rights; and so on. It is similar with the question of our ability to control our fates.

Parents of the post–World War II baby boomers in America tended to believe that things just happened to a person from the outside world. People of my parents' generation often seemed blind to their own role in producing the forces that beset them. If a relationship went badly, the other person was seen as just behaving oddly. If a child had a behavior problem, there was little inclination to think in terms of the family system. If one's health deteriorated, one thought in terms of germs and of the drugs to counter them, while giving little thought to how emotional stresses might have bred the vulnerability to illness.

Then, in the late 1960s and early 1970s, their children's generation began to create a corrective, more holistic vision of reality. This vision, unfortunately, had reactive and excessive features of its own. It became one of the defects of New Age thinking to carry to extremes the idea that we create our own reality.

I have encountered this excess several times, and it has always troubled me. In the early 1970s, when I taught at Prescott College in Prescott, Arizona, some of my students were exponents of something called Silva Mind Control. I recall exploring with these students the implications of their adopted belief system, and having them assert—in response to my probing question—that those who died in the concentration camps had brought that fate upon themselves. There was no need to adduce any evidence for this proposition; it simply had to be that way. All those millions—whole families, whole communities—effecting their own destruction.

Another occasion was in the late 1970s when I was frustrated in my effort to get my work published. My disappointment was compounded when someone who was otherwise unfailingly supportive subjected me to "blame the victim" assumptions of the same sort. He thought my work important, so there could be no other explanation of my not being granted what I deserved than this: I must be unconsciously defeating myself. I offered to show my friend my cover letters to see if he could discern how I was subtly producing the rejections I thought I didn't want. Or did he think that my means of influencing publishers was telepathic? No mechanism was ever identified.

Subsequently, when I was a published author who nonetheless had to struggle to survive economically, on various occasions I was told by sundry New Age friends and acquaintances that wealth could easily be mine. We get, it was explained, whatever we put out to the cosmos that we want. The key to my financial success was not the obvious course of changing my line of work, but rather learning to align my thoughts correctly. If I could practice the right kind of "abundance" consciousness, material abundance would naturally and automatically come flowing in. If I assumed the right spiritual posture, I could stop worrying about keeping a roof over the heads of my children.

"He alone will die who wishes to die, to whom life is intolerable," wrote the psychoanalyst George Groddeck.[11] (Groddeck was speaking not of all death, but specifically of that from tuberculosis.) I can just picture some poor soul hearing this and, though coughing his lungs out, rousing himself sufficiently to punch Groddeck in the nose.

QUARANTINE: THE DIVIDED WORLDS OF THE HEALTHY AND THE SICK

After all my thinking and reading, I found myself still hesitant to embark on a book project growing out of my illness. In the back of my mind, I discovered, was the fear of going public as a Sick Person. I feared somehow being discredited. This frailty, I imagined, would be seen as a lapse, a defect that would diminish my standing to speak—or to have spoken—on other matters that face us as a society. In my mind, it was as if the confession of illness would undermine the authority of my other works—the way Heidegger's dishonorable connection with the Nazis detracts, in many people's minds, from the authority of his philosophy.

I wondered, does this fear have any basis? As my brother, Ed, says: on the one hand, yes and no. The feeling of shame underlying this fear reflected in part my own prejudices about what constitutes a person's worth. But that sense of shame also corresponded with something real about the attitudes that exist in the world: a stigmatization of the ill. I have practiced it, and I have experienced it. Would I feel comfortable to portray myself in this decline even if I could not say, at the end, that in the final act of my drama I rose from the grave?

Most people would rather be spared the spectacle of the diseased and infirm. Keep away! Some of this reaction is clearly adaptive. Contagion is a factor in many diseases, and shunning contact with the diseased makes one's own survival more likely. If the smell of dead and putrid flesh is repulsive, if disgust is a natural response to the smell of human excrement, perhaps it is because too close a communion with such decadent matter can threaten our own health. (If our industrial civilization lasted for eons, would carbon monoxide cease to be odorless to human beings?) But there is more going on. We tell the sick not just to keep away, but also to keep out of sight.

In their touching book *Gramp,* Mark and Dan Jury document in words and pictures the decline into senility and eventual death of their beloved grandfather. One scene depicts the occasion when they took the demented but still good-natured old man to a local carnival. He encounters people he had long known, and in conversation with them reveals his belief that his own mother—in reality dead for several decades—is alive and somewhere nearby. After exchanging some pleasantries, his interlocutors take their leave. Later, say the Jurys, they learned that some of the people "thought it 'disgusting that they drag [the grandfather] out in public in the condition he's in.' "[12]

Shame on you.

Hester's scarlet letter, the yellow Star of David sewn onto the sleeve of a Nazi concentration camp victim, the dunce cap forced onto the heads of intellectuals during the Chinese Cultural Revolution's public humiliations: these are the images employed by Arthur Kleinman to portray how powerfully some diseases in our culture stigmatize their victims. He is talking here not about contagions, but about diseases that are frightening to us purely because they make their victims deviate from normal functioning, form, and movement—problems such as cerebral palsy, epilepsy, mental retardation, and other "disfiguring and crippling afflictions."[13]

Of course we are attracted to the healthy and energetic, and repelled by the wizened and deformed. It is hardly a coincidence that when the purveyors of cigarettes wish to persuade us to smoke, they put their butts in the hands of young and lively models, or that when the American Cancer Society or American Lung Association create a poster to persuade us to avoid the smoking addiction, they depict a shriveled, sickly older person in the grip of the habit.

We are wired to be turned on by health because our wiring is dictated by the demands of life, crafted over eons of selection choosing between the quick and the dead, and health is the blossom of life. Conversely, we are programmed to find disease, deformity, and death repulsive for the same reason.

Aside from the occasional saint inclined to kiss and bathe the leper, most of us choose flesh in a different state of repair for our kisses. Sexual attractiveness is a powerful force in the human animal, and while tastes are certainly influenced by culture, cross-cultural evidence suggests that the criteria for beauty are in large measure part of our inborn makeup. In a given population, the beautiful features appear to be the norm: for example, the most beautiful nose will be the one that is neither shorter nor longer, wider nor narrower than average. Regular, average features and proportions, smooth and graceful movements, a vigor—all are signs of a well-functioning specimen falling within the time-proven range of specifications for a given gene pool. One look at such evidence, and we feel the urge to combine one of our germ cells with one from that other person, and thus to wager our genetic future on that throw of the chromosomal dice.

Thus it is particularly heartrending to read of the distress of young people struck, before they have had a chance to create their new families, with conditions that sabotage their attractiveness. There is the voice of the young woman who, to save her life, must have a colostomy but then must bear the stigma and wonder what kind of future she will be able to have. And Moira Griffin shares openly her anguish at being transformed by her disease from an attractive young woman into one whom many men regard as auto-matically disqualified.

The healthy have many possible reasons for wishing to put dis-tance between themselves and the ill. But one of the most power-ful, though least acknowledged, is the threat the ill represent simply by their demonstrating the inherent vulnerability of the human condition. One way to avoid this unwelcome reminder is simply to keep away from those people who embody one's undesirable possi-ble—or inevitable—future. Because of my own unhappy sense near the inception of this project that I was doomed to long outlast the vital powers that I had most valued in myself, I was drawn to the question of how star athletes cope with their passage—only mid-way through their life span—to the far side of their prime and glory. My inquiry led me to talk with a psychologist who has done considerable research into the lives of retired professional football players. The psychologist, Dr. Anthony Bober of Irvine, California, relayed to me what retired football players had told him: once you leave the game, active players don't want to affiliate with you. For the men still playing, Bober told me, the retired player is a reminder of their vulnerability, that their careers will not continue forever.[14]

When we can't avoid unwelcome reminders of this kind, we find other ways to distance ourselves from those who incarnate a future we don't want to contemplate. In her book *The Private Worlds of Dying Children,* for example, Myra Bluebond-Langner describes the way children newly diagnosed with leukemia talk about those children on the leukemia ward whom they had known and who had died of the disease: they would accentuate the ways they were different from whatever child had died.[15] Moira Griffin describes a similar defensive strategy. When she was still in the initial stages of coming to terms with her multiple sclerosis, she met a woman with a more advanced case of the disease. During their conversation, the woman had manifested some bizarre symptoms and described others. Griffin became so agitated that, at the end of the meeting, "I dashed away. I felt wild. There was nothing about her that was like me—*nothing.*"[16]

Griffin confesses that she began to hate the woman whose MS so terrified her. Where there is fear, hostility is usually not far away. Just as there is a punitive and not just explanatory element in the "blame the victim" approach I described earlier, so also does antagonism help those who are defending themselves against their fears to distance themselves from those whose plight is too close for comfort. Barbara Sourkes, in her book *The Deepening Shade: The Psychological Aspects of Life-Threatening Illness,* describes a similar mechanism at work among a group of health professionals dealing with a patient whose similarity to themselves frightened them. The case involved a young nursing student who was suddenly diagnosed as having cancer, and was compelled to undergo a hasty amputation. Subsequently, she complained that the nurses were avoiding her and were hostile to her requests for pain medication. Eventually, the nurses were helped to confront what Sourkes calls "their difficulty in witnessing someone *so like themselves* go through such devastation. The woman's requests for pain medication reminded the nurses of her anguish, and—by identification—of their own vulnerability."[17]

The gap between the experience of one whose life is working well and one who is racked with agony can seem vast. To recognize that you might easily fall from the one to the other is like standing unprotected at the edge of a chasm. It is entirely understandable that those among us fortunate—or, as they might see it, virtuous, or favored, or special—enough to stand at one of life's higher places would wish to erect whatever kinds of barriers (real or illusory) can keep that sense of vulnerability at bay. Even if those barriers tend to quarantine off the less fortunate among their brothers and sisters.

BENEATH IT ALL THERE IS NO BOTTOM

The trolley took me to the foot of the hill on which sat the hospital where my father lay in pain. The good news was that he at last knew the cause of his pain. The bad news was that the cause— Hodgkin's disease eating at his bones—was also killing him. *"Kyrie Eleison,"* I sang quietly, fervently, to myself as I climbed the hill to New England Baptist Hospital. Lord have mercy upon us. I was not a believer, but still my song was a prayer. As a member of a high school choir I had sung Ralph Vaughan Williams's *Mass,* and now on this spring day in my freshman year in college I made the music the means for my entreaty to . . . to what I didn't know. Would my father live or die? In my personal cosmos, this question was so momentous that my rationally held belief that we are exposed to mere chance was overwhelmed by a feeling, welling up from deep within me, that something must decide our fate on some basis appropriate to the lives at stake. So I poured out my heart through my voice so that my feelings might weigh in the scales of reckoning. Lord have mercy on us.

The next best thing to believing you are in control of your fate is to believe that your future is being governed by outside forces that are entirely trustworthy. The power of self-determination is a gratifying feeling of an adult sort. But to see the cosmos as ruled by a being, or by an order, that is at once wise and good and powerful— that is to feel ensconced in the home of an ideal parent.

Sometimes the two kinds of reassuring belief systems are structurally indistinguishable. Betty Rollin's mother believed that the natural order of cause and effect guaranteed that if she ate impeccably she could not get cancer. Other people may believe that if they follow faithfully in the path of the righteous, God will spare them any terrible misfortune. The ideal parent in such a cosmic system reliably metes out good and bad in return for good and bad conduct. Eating broccoli can be another form of righteous-ness.

Both these systems of belief give reassurance to the fortunate among us, but both systems can be maintained only at the expense of the unfortunate. The precise nature of the causality may differ, but the effect of blaming the victim is the same. The naturalistic system of a Dr. Siegel might posit that if you have developed can-cer, your outlook must not have been loving enough. In a religious system, a similarly well-intentioned bystander might tell the af-flicted: you must have sinned.

In Esther Goshen-Gottstein's book about her husband Moshe's near-miraculous recovery from the deep coma he fell into after heart surgery, she relates a brief exchange that neatly illustrates some of the dynamics of this interpretive system. In the waiting room of a hospital near her home in Israel, where her husband was lying comatose, Goshen-Gottstein tells a man about her husband's crisis. The coma had already lasted three weeks, and the doctors did not expect him ever to emerge from it. In a good-faith effort to be helpful, the man in the waiting room, an orthodox Jew, suggests that she should check the texts of her mezuzot (scrolls placed by observant Jews in their doorways); perhaps a flaw in one might underlie their family catastrophe. Clearly it is reassuring to this orthodox man to believe that correctly following observance will bring safety. His propounding of that belief, however, drives a wedge between himself and the woman he is trying, as he would see it, to help. "I resented his simplistic faith," Goshen-Gottstein wrote, "which implied a connection between Moshe's coma and our failure to observe a religious precept flawlessly."[18]

Why would God allow disaster to befall the righteous? This problem is at the heart of a book that received a good deal of attention some years back: Rabbi Harold Kushner's *When Bad Things Happen to Good People*. I had heard of this book for years, and imagined—due, I now surmise, to some snobbish reflex—that a book so popular, and with so simpleminded a title, must be glib and insubstantial. Finally reading it for this project, when my own health and intellectual investigations led me to it, I was surprised and delighted to discover that it is really an admirable piece of work, full of humanity and intelligence.

As one might expect in a book written by a rabbi about "when bad things happen to good people," Kushner looks carefully at the Book of Job. Kushner comments on the reaction of Job's friends to seeing such a righteous man afflicted with a series of disasters. They face the dilemma, Kushner writes, of believing three things to be true: that Job is a good and deserving man, that God is all-powerful, and that God is all-good. Any two of these are compatible, but all three together are not. So Job's friends take what I would call the expedient course: they sacrifice Job. They react just like many in our own society do to the chronically ill, saying, in the words of Moira Griffin: "Surely you did something to bring this on yourself." About Job's friends' telling him that he must somehow deserve the affliction he is undergoing, Rabbi Kushner writes: "To say that everything works out in God's world may be comforting to the casual bystander, but it is an insult to the bereaved and the unfortunate."[19]

But even if we were all to agree that Job, Moira Griffin—and my father—were all good people undeserving of disaster, surely their fates must be fitting and right, in the service of some benign plan. Or so many people will assert when they employ another, less moralistic and hence less divisive, form taken by the (usually) comforting religious belief that all is as it should be. We move here from the notion of suffering as deserved punishment to the idea that events that appear bad are really good and useful parts of some larger picture. "God moves in mysterious ways his wonders to perform," as people often say. Preserving this comforting belief at least does not require us to scapegoat the sufferer. But this view is also, unfortunately, less comforting because it provides no assurance that any degree of virtue will protect one from harm. Unprotected from suffering, we find comfort in the belief that at least our suffering must have a meaning and purpose. A child with cystic fibrosis, whose account is one chapter in Jill Krementz's *How It Feels to Fight for Your Life,* says, "I have faith there is a reason I have this disease. God didn't just draw my name out of a hat."[20] The husband of a woman with multiple sclerosis tells his wife: "You have to believe that if God wants you to get better, you will get better, and if He doesn't, there has to be some purpose to it."[21]

Another book provides Kushner a text with which to explore this "God's plan" way of explaining life's disasters: Thornton Wilder's *The Bridge of San Luis Rey.* At the beginning of this short novel, a bridge collapses, killing a handful of unrelated travelers who were on the bridge at that fateful moment. Troubled by witnessing this accident, a priest sets out to investigate. He discovers that in each case it proved to be a fitting moment for the life to end.

Kushner doesn't buy this God's plan explanation. In works of fiction, where there is indeed an omnipotent planning mind overseeing the composition of events, tragedies may indeed fall at just the appropriate moment on just the appropriate person, but, Kushner maintains, "real life is not all that neat."[22] He thinks of airline crashes, in which two hundred and fifty people are instantaneously snuffed out. Doesn't it defy credulity to suppose that all these people's lives were somehow ripe for termination?

For Kushner, these questions are not mere chatter; his inquiry grows out of the guts of his own life. The book is the fruit of Kushner's own long struggle, as a man of faith, to come to terms with a painful personal tragedy: the birth of a son with a congenital defect that would condemn him to an abbreviated life filled with great physical suffering. Kushner understands Job's pain firsthand, and he also knows Job's anger.

What kind of God would inflict such suffering on the innocent, he wonders, regardless of how great His Big Plan might be? Kushner could not excuse such a God. "If a human artist or employer made children suffer so that something immensely impressive or valuable would come to pass, we would put him in prison."[23]

Faced with the problem of those three beliefs, of which one must be sacrificed, Kushner chooses a solution different from that elected by Job's friends. He concurs with them in rejecting the idea of God as a criminal—one who willfully torments the innocent—but unlike them he will not blame the victim. Kushner cannot conceive how his sweet and much-loved son deserved such suffering. Therefore, he concludes, God must not be all-powerful. My father took the third approach: after accidentally dismembering a frog with a lawnmower, my father—a lifelong agnostic in the painful throes of his own terminal cancer—spent some days filled with fury about the cruelty of God.

Kushner proposes that we see God as unable to command the fall of every sparrow, as unable to script the flow of all events. The realm of causality, he suggests, operates free from the reigning hand of an all-powerful governor. In the words of the popular bumper sticker, "Shit happens." God's part in the drama of our suffering, says Kushner, is not to inflict pain but to strengthen and console us in our dealing with it. I see this as a shift in parental imagery: no longer the paternal ruler, but rather the maternal comforter.

It remains unclear in Kushner's account on what evidence he concludes that God enters into our coping process to comfort or to fortify us. Kushner is not a proponent of that belief according to which God gives us no more than we are capable of bearing, for he recognizes that some people are broken by the burden of grief that life imposes on them. Nor does Kushner explain why a God who can make an appearance as helper in the suffering of countless individuals would not have the further capability of managing events. It seems to me that he is struggling to maintain as much of the biblical image of a personal deity as possible, and ends up preserving more of it than—to me, at least—the evidence alone suggests. Nonetheless, I deeply admire the intellectual and moral courage that Kushner shows in allowing, as far as he does, his fundamental beliefs to be transformed under the impact of his own life experiences.

In the three and a half years my father had left to live after the crisis that brought him to New England Baptist Hospital, he wrestled with the Book of Job. I don't think he ever found a satisfying way to come to terms with the excruciating pain that, from time to time, sang through his body—no way, that is, of finding meaning in it.

My father suffered bravely, which is to say he did not compel those of us who loved him to suffer with him. But from the loss of him there was no such protection. Even as I told myself that there need be no answer to the question, "Why?" there was a part of me that insisted on asking it. What did it *mean* that my father—such a fine man—had not been allowed to live out the fullness of his days? Why had his life story ended so soon, and with such pain?

I found then—and I can find now—no satisfactory answers to such questions. I believe in a sacred dimension, as several of my earlier works attest. And I believe in the great power of that dimension to enter into our lives and affect us in profound ways. But I cannot see that the sacred—or God—operates in such a way that we are assured that events either will be fair or that they will serve a good purpose.

When I reached the age at which my father had fought his losing battle with cancer, I found myself engaged in my own battle for health. My pain did not compare with his, and there was no reason to think that my life was in jeopardy as his had been. But nonetheless I, too, had been "struck down in the prime of life." And I, too, felt a need to find the "meaning" of it.

Even in the absence of a belief in a providential God to compose our lives in accordance with merit, or with some divine plan serving divine purposes, I found a fundamental resistance—even a cognitive incapacity—to wrapping my mind around the idea that . . . I was going to say, "We are the playthings of Chance," but even that locution implies that there is something out there playing with us. The uncomputable idea, rather, is that "Shit just happens." That the Lisbon earthquake had nothing to do with the sins of the believers. That the earth might be wiped out by some asteroid streaking in from the heavens for no reason that has anything to do with the terms and values that define how we live our lives.

When we watch a movie, we can often sense where things are heading. Plots unfold according to a logic that weaves meaning. For example, pride cometh before a fall in *Oedipus,* thus showing the *hubris* in the idea that man is the measure of all things. The prayers of innocent children are answered in *Angels in the Outfield.* Our narratives are orchestrations of meaning. We know that there is no way that, right in the middle of the movie, our main character is going to carelessly step off the curb in front of a taxi and be killed.

Even while I see no evidence to suggest that human events are scripted by a great Playwright, I also observe that I cannot grasp that my life should not have the same protections as the movie character on the curb in the middle of the movie. Crouched over the toilet where the meal that would not go down right has, by my invitation, just come back up, I wonder: how can it be that my life—the life of the great Me—has come to this? This is not the way my life is supposed to be! I protest. My life is supposed to be a Great Quest. This crap is just an interruption of the drama. It just gets in the way of my life taking the form it's supposed to: this isn't really part of the movie about Schmookler's life, but just some interference from the inability of the tape to track properly. Where can I get another copy of the tape?

Of course, there is no other tape. There is no guarantee that my life, or anyone else's, will track a course one finds fitting.

I recall a scene with my family. It is a good morning, meaning that my head is clear and my heart is strong enough to be open. I'm glad of the timing, having an open heart on this day when all five of us—April and Aaron and Terra and Nathaniel and I—will be together the whole day, driving to Virginia Beach for the holidays. I feel my love for all these beautiful creatures that make up my family; blessed to be part of this family picture.

Then I think of the road ahead, all the holiday traffic moving at sixty-five miles per hour and more, and the thought goes through my mind: perhaps the unthinkable will happen; perhaps we'll be in an accident. But no! That part of me calls out which had sung the *Kyrie* on the way up that Boston hill. That wouldn't be fitting: especially for the kids, it isn't their time. They've got their whole lives ahead of them. They are too splendid to be cheated of life in that way. There is no way a car accident at this point could end it all.

Then I laugh at myself, bitterly. I've read the newspapers. Other families get wiped out. Were they any less cheated than we would be? I doubt it. I, too, don't buy *The Bridge of San Luis Rey*. Shit just happens.

One night years ago I had a dream that articulated well for me this somewhat unnerving vision of the nature of things. In this dream, a former teacher and mentor of mine sat down at the organ and announced that we would now play the cantata by Vivaldi, "Beneath It All There Is No Bottom." Upon reflection, I could see that it was fitting for him to appear in my dream in this role: this man was a person whose wisdom and depth of mind I respected, as I still do; he was a person by whom, at a crucial moment a few years earlier, I had felt betrayed and abandoned, a completely unexpected occurrence that felt very much like the bottom falling out of my life.

My experience since then, including the vicissitudes of my health, has often moved me to think appreciatively of the title of that fictitious work by Vivaldi. It captures well the startling—sometimes scary, sometimes invigorating—condition in which we all find ourselves as bundles of life upon this spinning speck of dust in this incomprehensibly immense universe.

CHAPTER 2

Living Posthumously

How One Deals with Loss

EUREKA!

I was sitting out on our deck with the sweep of our beautiful valley before me. But I was not moved. Or rather, I was moved only further toward despondency because the instrument of my being seemed unable to register the beauty of the sight. Like a camera with the lens cover left on. It felt as though some toxicity in my blood was out in full force, relentlessly suppressing my vitality. I breathed, my heart beat, my mind was clear (if listless)—but it was as though I was already dead.

The phrase keeps going through my mind: living posthumously.

This house on a ridge in Virginia's Shenandoah Valley was the fruit of a three-month, full-time search for a new place for us to live, a new life. There had been some evidence that where we lived—inside the Washington Beltway, in a damp little hollow, in a dark and moldy house—might have been an important factor in my difficulties. My downhill course seemed to begin around the time we had moved in. When I was away on longer trips, my condition seemed to improve. Sherry Rogers's tests had ascertained that my allergic sensitivity to molds was of near-record proportions. I had always seemed sensitive to pollution in the air. Why not try, as an experiment, some time in a very different place?

At the outset, the central idea was to find a place where the countryside was free of car exhaust and the house was clear of dust and mold. Soon, however, a different spirit began to animate the hunt. I was searching in an area defined by the arc of what could be reached from Washington or Baltimore within two hours. My two children from my first marriage had to be able to get back and forth between my house and their mother's, which was in Baltimore. My mother lived in Takoma Park—lived alone—and we needed to stay within easy visiting range of her. For those reasons, my dreams of returning to the mountains of the West—where my relationship to the land had once deepened my spiritual aliveness beyond anything I had experienced before or since—could not be acted upon. But the land within reach of those eastern cities, I discovered, had a spirit of their own that spoke to me. More and more, as I explored the mountains west of Gettysburg and the wetlands around the Chesapeake, the beauty of the land called out to me. Maybe not just the physical aspects of the air, but the spiritual aspects of my connection with the earth were essential to bringing me back to life. I recalled the spiritual void that was left in me when I moved from Prescott, Arizona, to the city—recalled how after a few months of grieving I had become used to the city, almost forgot what I was missing, and how that accommodation had entailed a hollowing out of my spiritual life. Maybe what had happened to me after a decade inside the Washington Beltway was the cumulative result of being so long cut off from a landscape that recharged my batteries. Maybe in my sickness I was like that pallid and bloated E.T. who needs to get out of this alien place to save his life.

My quest for a house, thus, gradually changed from a search for someplace clean to one for a spot whose beauty charged my spirit with a sense of the sacred.

When I started, my intention was to find a place to rent for half a year. But as the process became a spiritual quest, and as the criteria expanded and deepened to incorporate the need for a place where there was a there there, the impracticality of that idea became apparent. In an America where respect for the landscape has been all but obsolete among the builders of houses for the better part of a century, there were just not enough places that spoke to my spirit, and the places offered for rent were too few, for the rental market to offer much promise. So, after much deliberation and with much trepidation, April and I decided to consider actually buying a house. We imposed on ourselves the discipline that our total cost for housing could not exceed the rent we were then paying on the humble house we were renting in Silver Spring, Maryland, and then resumed the search. What had been intended as an experiment thus became a leap of faith.

That our leap took us to the mountains of Virginia was the result not of our prior decision, but of the way our search just happened to pan out. For three months I played a game of realty roulette that took me into various nooks and crannies of Pennsylvania, Maryland, West Virginia, and Virginia. We might have settled in any of those areas if the right place had been on the market at an affordable price. But it was here in the Shenandoah Valley that I finally found a spot where I could say, "This is the place." And what a place! Gardens and an orchard, a driveway sculpted sensitively along the curve of the hillside, and a view of several square miles of mountains and valley shaped not by the hand of our species so much as by the hand of the Creator, or at least by the forces of Nature. It was with great hope that I, now down to 135 pounds, moved the family and our belongings out to the mountains.

Now, a couple months after our arrival, the air was clear, but the spirit was still clouded. All that beauty, but what was it worth to me if my spirit could not resonate with it. Even the grandest feast cannot nourish a dead man.

THE AUTHOR'S REMAINS

I was still living posthumously.

Those words came to me on the day of that first summer when I received a telephone call from a kind couple who had succeeded— or so they thought—in tracking down the author of *The Parable of the Tribes.* It was the kind of call that ordinarily would have been deeply heartening to me. The book had changed the way they see the world, added a fourth dimension to it, solved mysteries—just the sort of experience I had sought to impart, to do for others what that vision had done for me. And they wanted to come out here to meet and talk with the author.

Of course I said yes, but I had the uneasy feeling I was in some way defrauding them. Underlying that feeling, I found, was the sense that I'm not the author of that book. Or rather, I felt that I was, in some way, only what was left of him after his mysterious demise. I saw their trip as a pilgrimage to the graveside of some person whose work one has appreciated. But can one say that one has visited Ben Franklin in Philadelphia, or Charles Dickens in England, or Elvis in Memphis?

"You are welcome to come," I felt I should have told them, "if it would be worth your while to visit the author's remains."

LOSS OF SOUL

I was talking on the phone with my brother, Ed. He's often the one I turn to when I am wrestling with life's deeper issues. As different as we are, we two brothers also make up together a rather deep culture of two, the offspring of Jacob and Pauline Schmookler. We speak the same language, and we can readily fly together through realms of meaning that, with other people, might take the equivalent of a lot of pointing and gesturing to begin to reach.

"I feel like my soul has leaked out," I told him. "It all makes me think this soul idea is such an illusion. What kind of soul can it be if sometimes you have it and sometimes you don't? You believe in the soul?"

"Yeah, I do," he replied. "And I don't buy the notion that you don't have a soul. Feeling bad, even feeling empty, doesn't prove that the essence of you isn't there. Isn't it from your soul that you feel the anguish you do about being trapped in this cloud?"

"But what about April's father? What about a guy like him with Alzheimer's disease who is still alive but couldn't tell you who he is or that he is alive? What about these people whose bodies keep on ticking but seem to have no spirit left, no thinking or feeling like what defined them when they were healthy? Where is their soul—already off to heaven, or trapped in the body, incapable of manifesting itself?"

Ed hesitated. He's a thoughtful guy. "I think that even with someone who can't comb his hair, or take a leak in the right place—even with him, I think that his essence is still there, that there is still a human soul in that ruined body."

"I'm impressed that you think so, Ed, but I don't see it. Seems to me that, though we may have a soul, it's tied into our chemistry, into the soup and wires that make up our brain, and that there's nothing in our essence that can't be altered when that physical stuff gets messed up."

GO ON WITHOUT ME

"If I'm dead, what does that make April? A widow." That melancholy idea would come to me sometimes, and it saddened me deeply. Even in my darkened state, April's presence and my love for her was a big part of what brightness my life had. But the full human being that she had chosen to spend her life with, I believed, had disappeared. She didn't have what she had bargained for. The old vows talk about for better or worse, in sickness and in health. But if I really love April, I figured, I wouldn't hold her to that. She had a right to a life where her mate didn't hold her back.

It was a long while before I spoke to April about these thoughts. Then, one night when we were out for a walk along the wooded streets in our neighborhood in Silver Spring, the subject came up. I was expressing my frustration—was she tired of having to hear so often of my distress?—that my malady was one problem from which I couldn't separate myself. Unlike having a bad job, say, there was no getting away from it.

"But that's not true for you, April," I told her. "Your life and mine are entwined—but not inseparable." I stopped and faced her, taking both her hands in mine. "You know those scenes in the movies where a couple of people are trying to escape over the mountain from the pursuing Nazis? How one of them gets shot and falls, and his comrade stops by his side to try to help him? The guy always tells his friend to go for it. No point in them both losing their lives. That's what I want to say to you, April. If being married to me is costing you your life—and it seems to me it must be— you don't have to stay here by me. I want you to be free to go for it. I don't want you to have to live the life of a widow, with me occupying a position in your life that there's not enough of me to really fill."

April is not one of those tearful women, which makes my life easier, though sometimes I miss that particular form of expressiveness—a woman's tears being sometimes wonderfully moving for a man like me who does not cry easily. But she does have special eyes. I'd spoken of them in the vows I had composed for our wedding, recalling the first moment I saw her above Pierce Mill in Rock Creek Park. "Your face shone at me like a beacon," I said at our wedding gathering, "your eyes like an open blue sky." She has the eyes of someone who is kind and who tells the truth. She looked at me now as we stood together under the streetlight, and I wondered how kindness and truth would be combined when she spoke next.

She put her hands gently on my shoulders, and then turned her head and rested it against my chest. "I'm sorry you're suffering, Andy. But I'm not a widow. I love our life together. It would be great if you felt better, but just as you are you're the one I want to be married to."

But what about me always pooping out when we go biking? What about the dampening of her lover's animal spirits? What about the hassle of our having this part-time job of taking care of me? Why should you have to live the rest of your life beside a goddamn cloud?

"Some things may have changed," April said, "but in all the essential ways you're still the man I fell in love with."

"I'm glad you're still in touch with the guy. Next time you see him, would you tell him to come see me?"

THE DEATHS IN LIFE

"Cowards die many times before their deaths," says Shakespeare's Caesar. "The valiant never taste of death but once."[1] I'm not so sure of that. In the course of life, each of us inevitably will suffer many losses, and every kind of loss is experienced as a kind of death.

The self is a multifaceted entity. Our humanity depends upon our being able to invest our selves in people beyond our own individual boundaries. What one loves becomes as if part of one's own living tissue. To lose one's beloved is as if, in some measure, one has died oneself.

When, in the *Book of Roland,* Gawain recognizes his dead brother, "his legs gave way, his heart failed, and he fell as if dead." At Ronceveaux, on seeing his good men slain, Charlemagne declares, "I wish no more to live."[2]

The closer the relationship, the more like a death is the experience of bereavement. Not every loss of a loved one is through actual biological death. In nineteenth-century Ireland, the departure of family members for America was a frequent occurrence, and it generally meant that those who left would never be seen again. The families held what was called an "American wake" for their children leaving for a new life overseas.[3]

There is now a literature on the subject of bereavement, and it represents the insight that each kind of loss is in some experiential way equivalent to every other kind. Thus the experiences of widowhood, of the loss of a home, of amputation, are all understood in the same conceptual rubric.[4]

Betty Rollin's first book is about the loss of a part of her body. The reason was cancer, and the part removed was a breast. For her, as a young and attractive woman, a good deal of her self was invested in her dearly departed left breast. As she tries to explain the experience, she reaches for an analogy from another kind of bereavement: "I am like a widow who doesn't get it at first. Then she wakes up the next morning and the place next to her on the bed is empty, the sheets still tucked in on the other side, the pillow high and plumped, and she gets it then. I look at the empty place on my body and I get it, too. . . . One remembers the dead fondly. . . . I remember my left breast with love, real love."[5]

Not only does death come for us all, but it comes many times in many forms. The challenge of learning how to live posthumously is thus one that, in varying degrees and in diverse ways, we all have to meet in the course of our life span.

SHADOW OF MY FORMER SELF

I felt as if I'd been robbed by a thief who somehow knew just where my valuables were hidden. I wouldn't have minded so much giving up my wallet and watch, but this thief seemed to have known where the jewels were kept.

On the way to basketball one night with my friend Bob Danforth, I said, in response to his inquiry, yeah, my work is going fine. I can still do it. But it's like what I imagine it would be for Michael Jordan to play basketball with a seventy-five-pound vest on. He'd still be playing the game, but he wouldn't be Michael Jordan. Not at least the Air Jordan that had made him special.

In my book *Fool's Gold,* I used the metaphor of a piano to represent the human organism, and the vibration of our strings as our capacity to respond to the spectrum of our experience. A blanket thrown across those strings I used as an image for an impairment of that capacity. Later, that image came to my mind, painfully, out of the intermittent damping of my own ability to register the wonderment of human life.

It's not enough to think thoughts, I discovered. The deeper resonances are needed to make them meaningful. The "Wow" of wonderment and the "Aha" of excitement at my own insights turned out to be necessary to fuel the engines of my creativity.

What becomes of the calling of a "visionary," I wondered, when moving the eyes is like lifting weights. I've always liked the line, "I lift up mine eyes to the mountains, from whence cometh my help." But now I felt strained to raise my eyes. And helpless.

Some aspects of oneself are more central than others. When I started playing basketball again at forty, after a ten-year retirement, the only major difference I noticed in my body became clear while the team was doing layup drills: when I jumped up to put the ball onto the backboard, I hardly left the ground. Compared to the layup I used to shoot when I was in high school, it was an entirely new shot I had to learn now. I felt sorry to discover that my spring had sprung, but for a "social thinker" in his forties, it was a loss on which I did not have to spend much grieving.

But the recurrent general loss of energy and of a more subtle but still vital spiritual spark is different. My life was structured around my ability at moments to encompass the human situation in a deeper and more comprehensive way than my usual perspective. What those moments are like is not easy to describe, though I can say that all my previous books stand essentially as monuments to such occurrences. At those times, I feel that I am no longer bound by the confines of my small self, that my consciousness expands to take in the world, that my vision encompasses some of the large flows of energy and structure through the time and space of history, that my normally thin repertoire of experience could fatten itself through identification with the points of view and feelings of others very different from me. And from all this, I would be rewarded by an inner sense of richness and excitement.

At a certain point, I began to fear that those spiritual and intellectual expanses would henceforth be forever closed to me. My malady seemed to be condemning me to the prison of an ever-narrowing self and range of response. I grieved.

There is a Buddhist story of a woman who is beside herself with grief at the death of her son, and is comforted only after she is sent on a mission to get a mustard seed from whatever house she can locate that has been untouched by death. Her efforts, while failing of course to bring her son back to life, do bring her the discovery that her loss is an inescapable part of the human condition, and in this she finds consolation.

I see myself as having been like this woman. Like her, I found my loss unbearable: this should not happen to me. Like her, I have been consoled to some degree to recognize that I am not unique in my loss.

I set out to explore the experience of others who are compelled to outlive their special gifts, who lose what they had formed their identity around well before they must give up life itself. Athletes, for example, as mentioned earlier. I was moved to read about the professional football player who, because of injuries sustained during his playing career, now struggles to go up and down stairs.[6] Here is a man who, from the time of his earliest youth, enjoyed the heroic status our society confers on those with exceptional physical gifts; and now even the normal movements of daily life strain his capacities. How do such men cope with so great a fall so early in life?

Many athletes spend a good deal of their lives in the unhappy twilight of the has-been. Arnold Beisser, in his book *Flying Without Wings,* writes about the men, frequently to be found in bars drowning their sorrows, who speak with enthusiasm only about their athletic glories long past. "It is as though life stopped with the end of the athletic career," Beisser says.[7] (Beisser himself knows what it is like to live posthumously, and to have to create a new basis for life: his book is an autobiographical account of his sudden encounter with catastrophic loss. A hot-shot tennis player with a newly issued medical degree, Beisser was suddenly struck down in his twenties with a case of polio that put him in an iron lung for a long spell and that left him permanently paralyzed.

What athletic prowess is to many a young man, great physical beauty is for many young women. It is a key to a strong and positive identity, but it gives out well before the life span is complete. Two centuries ago, Samuel Johnson spoke to the plight of fading beauties for whom "age begins early, and very often lasts long." From the time that their bloom begins to wilt, "all which gave them joy vanishes from about them; they hear the praises bestowed on others, which used to swell their bosoms with exaltation."[8]

A reader of *The Sun* magazine addressed the pain of losing sexual attractiveness barely halfway through life. Answering the invitation from the magazine to its readers to write about aging, this woman, who withheld her name, wrote, "Young women *shine* with the fox fire of fertility." She had enjoyed the power that comes from this fire, but now, approaching menopause, "men sniff at me," she says, "and turn away."[9]

The eventual fading of beauty is inevitable, but illness can hasten the process. Moira Griffin recounts the story of her walking one day when her disease (MS) had changed her gait from "normal to spastic." She passed an old man who previously, when she was looking good, made lewd remarks to her as she walked past. This time, as she limped by,

> he said gently, "Angel, how ya doin?"
> I suppose I should have felt "See, he's not so bad." But instead I had to hold back the tears—he pitied me! A line from a poem I wrote in college went round and round in my head: sexless as an angel. Sexless as an angel.[10]

An old identity dies, through the ravages of disease or through the sheer passage of time, while life itself goes on. Sometimes, the disruption and the grief from the loss are so great that the continuation of life seems no blessing.

Several years ago, in an exploration of how the warrior spirit works in our civilization, I spoke about how some warriors have been so heavily identified with their honor that a life without it is virtually inconceivable.[11] As Shakespeare's Anthony puts it, "If I lose my honor, I lose myself" and his Richard II, "My honor is my life." If this ideal part of myself (my honor) is the heart of my identity, I would not wish to live without it. Similarly with other aspects of oneself that are bound together with the essence of one's sense of oneself: the loss of that part will feel like a loss of the whole.

In a document called the Heiligenstadt testament, Beethoven expresses his anguish about his loss of hearing. He laments that his disability cripples "the *one sense* that should be perfect to a higher degree in me than in others, the one sense which I once possessed in the highest perfection, a perfection that few others of my profession have ever possessed."[12] The despair he felt when someone could hear a shepherd singing, while he himself could hear nothing, is so great that "it would have needed little for me to put an end to my life." While Beethoven decides to remain alive in order to fulfill as much as possible of his artistic destiny, if death comes he will be content, "for will it not free me from a condition of endless suffering?"[13]

In their book *Building a New Dream,* Maurer and Strasberg tell of a young man confined to a wheelchair in the wake of a serious motorcycle accident. "They said he was lucky to survive, but now a year later he was quite convinced he would have been luckier dead."[14] In a modern equivalent of turning toward the wall, this man spent his days watching television, gaining weight, and not returning calls from friends, who liked to do things in which he now felt himself incapable of joining.

Every one of us has an identity, and we each have powers that are important to us, whether they are extraordinary in the great scheme of things or not. To rise from the grave of an old self with a new and satisfying identity is no easy task.

SMALL COMFORT

When we made the move to the mountains, two books of my series on the materialism of our civilization were being published, but one important piece of the whole remained to be drawn. But I no longer felt able to write it.

Why is it, I asked at the outset of that project, that though we are so rich by any historical standard, we are still so hungry for more? An important part of the answer, I felt, lies in the dynamics of our systems—in particular the inherent logic of the market economy and its power, over time, to shape a society and the values and motivations of its members. This part of my answer I had already articulated in *The Illusion of Choice: How the Market Economy Shapes Our Destiny* and *Fool's Gold: The Fate of Values in a World of Goods.*

It had been my plan to look next at the problem more directly from the inside, at the human scale: what makes us so discontent with what we have, so willing to sacrifice other sacred values in our lust for more of what we already possess in such abundance? *Filling a Sieve,* this book was to be called, and in it I was to delve into the psychological and spiritual bases for our insatiable appetite for material wealth.

As I stood on the deck of my new chalet home in the mountains, I considered where my work should go next. Our move was complete, the boxes cleared away, our new lives established. The move itself had been a real piece of work. But now it was time to return to the calling by which I usually justify my consumption of oxygen on this planet—my creative work.

Although I had promised my readers that *Filling a Sieve* was coming, and although I had already outlined that still-unwritten book in detail before I even began writing the first volume of the project, I felt in no position to speak to the world from that place now. For I was now learning from the inside something about the weakened state that helps engender our materialism.

The healthy human creature has access to deeper sources of nourishment; wounded and weakened, it is more apt to seek solace in the realm of material pleasures. Weakened now myself, I found that I was becoming more materialistic in my orientation. What disabled me was different from the kinds of wounding on which I was intending to focus. For me, for example, it was not a lack of nourishing relationships, as my family was just as I wished it to be. But I was not intact enough inside, at some fundamental level, to draw the sustenance from it that was available. Like a broken container—like a sieve—I could not hold the nectar. So, in some respects, it may amount to the same thing: unable to feel good at a deep level, I had an increased appetite for diversions and consolations.

As I thought about it, soothing myself in the waters of the hot tub at my new home, which I would never otherwise have obtained, save by inheriting it from a desperate seller in a buyer's real estate market, I realized that something else lodged still closer to the heart of it. *Comfort.* It is comfort for which my appetite had increased. Being beset by chronic discomfort had rearranged my strategic priorities. For those in pain, the most appealing thing imaginable might be a truly comfortable chair, or a hot soaking bath, or something soothing to drink. My new materialism seemed to be of this kind: I wanted comfort for my aching self, I wanted ease and convenience so that my dwindling reserves of energy would not be taxed too much, I wanted my nest feathered.

Now dried and dressed, reclining in my old La-Z-Boy, I thought that perhaps this is why the elderly so often seem so preoccupied with the material: physically depleted, with comfort and security hard to achieve, they turn their priorities toward the soft and sumptuous. These priorities drive a person deeper into the world of material goods.

If I ever returned to *Filling a Sieve* I'd have to look more deeply into this need for comfort, and how that might relate to some thoughts about the body I already intended to develop, according to which our materialism is a sign not of our being deeply connected and at home with our material dimension—in the body— but on the contrary of our being cut off from the roots of bodily pleasure.

But until I could recover my capacity for deeper spiritual nourishment, I would not tackle the book. From the vantage point of my unhealthy condition, I didn't feel able to contemplate these questions properly or to say what needed to be said.

PARADOXES OF IDENTITY, OR IS IT REALLY ME?

We live with time, through time, all the time, so it seems perfectly natural, entirely matter-of-fact. But time is really a strange riddle. Here's a little piece of what puzzles me.

We like to see continuities across time. For example, we celebrate anniversaries. America celebrated its bicentennial in 1976, regarding that year as special because two hundred years had passed since the nation's founding. If we had six fingers on each hand instead of five, we wouldn't have our bicentennial, or the duodecimal equivalent, until 288 years had gone by.

For that matter, how meaningful is the idea of a year? When we say, "On this day, in such-and-such a year, so-and-so was born," what does that mean? It means that the earth was in the same position in relation to the sun then as now. Given the reality of the earth's seasons, obviously the notion of an annual cycle is not entirely arbitrary. Yet the sun is itself in motion in our galaxy, and our galaxy is engaged in a slow but unceasing dance with the countless other galaxies. So, when we speak of "this day" in some other year, to some degree we are creating a fiction.

The Greek philosopher Heraclitus maintained that everything is in flux, that all is constantly changing. You can never step into the same river twice.

The changes that time and illness have wrought in me have brought Heraclitus's image of the changing river to my mind more than once. It is not only the river that changes each time one steps into it, but the one doing the stepping is also a different person with each step.

When a rose has faded, and its petals begin to drop off one by one, is it the same flower as the rose that not long before was so fresh and lovely in bloom?

One of my sons is now a young man, taller than I and old enough to drive. On the wall by our stairwell are pictures of the boy he was—the one-year-old crawling up to the polar bears' cage at the Tucson zoo, the six-year-old puffing out his chest in his Halloween Superman outfit with his shoes untied. I remember both those little boys, remember how it felt to carry each of them, sleeping, from the car to his bed. Of course, I know that there's more than just a name—Aaron—that constitutes the thread of continuity between those little boys and the adolescent who occasionally enjoys calling me "Shorty." But it also seems to me that the young man is a fundamentally different being from the boys that bore the same name.

A millennium ago, the Arab philosopher poet Ousama Ibn Mounkidh decried the ravages of age. "Marvel," he wrote, "also at a hand incapable of managing the kalam, after it has broken lances in the breasts of lions."[15] But is the hand that cannot manage the kalam the same hand that slew the lions?

Each stage of life seems to bring with it elements that are rather predictable. A two-year-old is likely to have at least as much in common with another two-year-old as with the five-year-old he or she will soon become, let alone the adult he or she will be later. The voices of old women sound as if they belong in the same flock. It is almost as though, as we pass through life, we flow into and out of membership in various discrete species.

Brody presents the idea that "good care" of the geriatric patient "includes asking him to bring in a photograph of himself when he was 'in his prime,' whatever that means to him, and giving that photo a prominent place in the medical chart."[16] I can understand the reasons for such a practice: a decrepit old person is under the care of people in a very different stage of life, and the picture might enable the caregivers better to recognize the human connection between themselves and the aged person they are attending; this recognition might enhance the quality of the care they give. But is this really a kind of trick, trying to get the caregivers to perceive the patient before them as a person who no longer exists?

The idea of the old photo in the medical chart, Brody says, "is that one is reminded that one is treating a person who has a life story."[17] To what extent is this kind of "story" a fiction, something that is made up, a product of our imagination? Do we cultivate the idea of an enduring identity because recognition of the ceaseless flux we embody would make us feel too precarious? To what extent are we fabricating a "momentary stay against confusion," finding it more comforting to see ourselves as solid like a rock of ages than to acknowledge our riverlike transformations in the unstoppable aging process?

The decline I suffered prompted me to take a second look at that old story of the movie star, whose career had declined some years back, accosted on the street by a former fan. "Didn't you used to be so-and-so?" the fan asks. The fan had always seemed foolish to me, as well as insensitive. But I became less sure he was foolish.

A couple years later, I had occasion to recognize myself, and it was doubly reassuring. Though at one level I was coming to terms with the possibility that this debilitated state may be the hand I'm stuck with playing, another part of the picture that I saw clearly was that I would stop my quest to restore my health only when I succeeded, or died, which ever came first. Didn't I used to be Andy Schmookler? Yeah, and I still am.

It was reassuring to recognize that my indomitable will endured, that some essential things about me did not change. And with that recognition came a clear answer to that occasional doubt I felt: Am I perhaps just making a mountain out of a molehill in this whole business? If my old fighting spirit is still there—the same one that enabled me in my prime to spend fourteen years (figuratively) hanging by my fingernails onto the side of a cliff in order to get *The Parable of the Tribes* written and into the world—anything that could slow me down and wear me down this much could be no molehill.

THE BLESSING AND CURSE OF MEMORY

I sat in the living room with April's father. His Alzheimer's had progressed to the point where he could not remember what he was saying well enough to finish a sentence heading in the same direction he had in mind when he started it. I'd never known this man before his mind started to vanish, but for a whole family that was now also mine, he was a man who had been at the center of their lives, a man with a playful wit and a love of music, and a man who had been for my April the source of the encouragement that had made her so brave in the world. For them, the sight of this man mindlessly folding and unfolding a newspaper he could no longer read, juxtaposed against a lifetime of memories, was a source of pain that I could only begin to imagine. Wrestling myself with the painful recollection of a lot of "used-to-bes," I thought: memory is a mixed blessing.

A boy with cystic fibrosis has a contentment he believes might have eluded him if he had memories of a healthier state. "I think in some ways I'm better off than some kids who get paralyzed or go blind all of a sudden. It's so much easier if you don't know what you're missing because you've never had it to begin with."[18]

Is such lack of memory a blessing, or is it better to have had a capacity and lost it than never to have had it at all?

One can be liberated from the burden of painful memories either by never having had the experience of something better or by having lost, along with the capacity, the memory of having ever possessed it. Oliver Sacks tells about his encounter with the man who appears in the title of his unusually thought-provoking book *The Man Who Mistook His Wife for a Hat*. At one point in their interview, Sacks encourages the man—a quite sophisticated and intelligent man he calls Dr. P.—to put on his shoes. It becomes clear, however, that the man thinks his foot is his shoe, and vice versa, and so the instruction to put on his shoe leads to a ludicrous display of incomprehension and incompetence. After trying to help Dr. P. understand what any healthy two-year-old already knows, Sacks "helped him on with his shoe (his foot), to avoid further complication." Dr. P. himself, Sacks further observes, "seemed untroubled, indifferent, maybe amused."[19] The condition itself seemed to bring with it a kind of anesthetic of unawareness that averted the pain of recognition of one's deteriorated state.

Alzheimer's disease is often harder on the families than on its immediate victims. While the families must witness the progressive disintegration and disappearance of a person they have loved, those afflicted with the disease are often themselves oblivious to their descent into oblivion.

That's the way it was with Charles Maxwell Moore, April's father, and his Alzheimer's. By the standards of that horrific disease, in his case that period was mercifully short between the first noticeable impairment of his mental faculties and his eventual death when the destruction of the central nervous system reached the life-sustaining functions. But "short" still means at least several years, and in all this time I am not aware of his ever having indicated a clear recognition that he was being stripped of his faculties, ever having asked "What's happening to me, why am I losing my wits, what is the nature of this disease, and what is my prognosis?" Instead, he seemed simply to endure, unaware, the progressive peeling away of the layers of his personhood, apparently never fully comprehending that something that had been there before was missing.

I watched this unawareness with some bewilderment. I could not conceive that any disease might similarly rob me of my faculties without my noticing and crying out some kind of "Stop! Thief!" as if the illness were some nimble-fingered pickpocket that can take one's valuables and leave its victim poorer but none the wiser.

Then there is the question of whether I would prefer to notice. It is not as though April's father was unperturbed, for the confusion that the disease inflicted was certainly accompanied by fear and frustration. But he seemed at least spared the pain of grieving his own demise. On the other hand, might not that grief be a meaningful part of the completion of one's life?

Philippe Ariès, in his magisterial study of the history of death in Western civilization, has noted a profound change from medieval times to the present in what is regarded as a desirable way to die. For the medieval European, the process of dying was important, a ritual of transition whose proper observance was indispensable. To die suddenly—struck down unawares—was an unspeakable calamity. But it is just such a death—abrupt, without warning: now you see it, now you don't—that people in contemporary society generally say they would prefer. For most of us, apparently, the idea of saying good-bye to all we have valued seems more painful and frightening than meaningful.

This question—of which is worse, to lose something invaluable and to feel its loss or to be witless that anything has slipped away—is one that Oliver Sacks ponders. He compares his own Dr. P. with Zazetsky, the patient of the famous Russian neurologist Luria, who was immortalized in the book *The Man with a Shattered World*. Luria describes Zazetsky as having "fought to regain his lost faculties with the indomitable tenacity of the damned," whereas, as Sacks said, Dr. P. "did not know what was lost, did not indeed know that anything was lost." Which leads Sacks to wonder "who was more tragic, or who was more damned—the man who knew it, or the man who did not?"[20]

My whole life, memory has been something that I've cherished and cultivated. Employing memory, I've always carried my past along with me like a well-supplied backpack. The overall trajectory of my work life in adulthood might be said to have been determined by a few crucial moments that I have kept before my mind's eye as guideposts and sources of inspiration. In this way, my investment in memory has been a great asset. I know a number of other people of my generation who had moments of epiphany that were swallowed up by the currents of their lives, disappearing traceless like a stone falling into a river. The potentiality of events that could have been transformative was forfeited by a failure to resurrect those experiences through the exercise of the power of memory.

But as I descended into my debilitation, I came to see that forgetting has its good points. One beautiful April day, when even the smell of lilacs left me unmoved, despite my remembering the nostalgic link between that fragrance and my first kiss, it hurt to notice how memory and desire went unmixed. If "it might have been" are the saddest words, "it used to be" cannot be far behind.

In Esther Goshen-Gottstein's account of her husband's disappearance into coma and his subsequent long and difficult regathering of his lost faculties, she identifies a point, sixteen weeks after her husband's surgery, when "his mental suffering increased." It was when he began to gain "insight into his state," which was one of gross motor and intellectual incompetence. "Don't you know what an idiot I am?" he asked in anguish. Here is a man formerly of great accomplishment and great pride, and he is tormented to recognize that the man who could take pride in accomplishment was no longer there. When a friend came in, he said, "Look at someone who has died."[21]

But memory can also dissolve over time, losing its substantiality and verisimilitude. One's old self, recalled, is not flesh and blood but a mere shadow of that former self. In the aftermath of catastrophe, the antediluvian time can seem just a misty fantasy. A realm of experience not recently visited can gradually become beyond imagining.

Another patient described by Sacks is a woman who, because of neurological damage, has lost her proprioceptive sense, that is, she lacks the most elemental sensations of her body and where it is in space. "If only I could feel!" she cries. "But I've forgotten what it's like." Memory fails, and the reality of the time before the loss seems less than real. "I *was* normal, wasn't I?" she asks Dr. Sacks. "I *did* move like everyone else?"[22]

To really remember in a full-bodied way—whether we judge such memory to be a blessing or a curse—is not always easy. It is difficult, for example, to remember one state of consciousness while held in the grip of another. Studies by psychological researchers have shown this: what you have learned in one state of consciousness you are much more able to recall when you are again in that state. I experience this frequently with dreams. Sometimes in one of my dreams, reference will be made to some event or symbol from another dream, long forgotten, that I dreamt years or decades ago. In my waking state, I would never have been able to retrieve that material. People report much the same from experiences with psychoactive drugs: frequently, with the return to normal awareness, even vivid and fascinating images and ideas will slip away (in the same way that most of us, upon awakening, drop our night's dreams into a sea of forgetfulness); then upon returning to the altered state by using the psychedelic substance again—even long after—the long-buried past experiences rise again into accessible memory.

Is this state-specificity of each set of memories a positive adaptation or is it an incidental by-product of our neurochemistry? I can imagine that there is some efficiency derived from storing memories so that they come back to us when, as it were, we revisit the same place. On the other hand, we can become maladaptively trapped when we are confined to a truncated portion of our total memory picture.

Something of this sort seems to happen, for example, with depression. When in a depressed frame of mind, one's retrospective glance through one's story is likely to yield a highly selective set of memories that yield a rather distorted portrait of the past. As one lapses into depression, or even just the blues, one is suddenly apt to recall easily—and only—all the other dark times. The resulting impression that "My life has always been miserable" not only compounds the misery of the moment, but it can also create a kind of black hole from which there is no ready escape. Our selective memory can thus be maladaptive, cutting us off from those parts of our past that might help us break out of the confines of an unwanted present.

Illness can bear with it its own state of consciousness, and seems capable, like depression, of generating its own selectivity of memory. A person long held in the grasp of a chronic illness may find it difficult to recall with any vividness that there had been any other way of living. Again, perhaps a positive and adaptive aspect of this can be conceived. Perhaps this tendency to forget what is very different from the present state can help us come to terms with that state: "This is life, so I might as well make the best of it." Perhaps too much cultivation of memory can make it more difficult to come to terms with unwelcome alterations of one's state of being.

But, on the other hand, memory can also be a very useful resource.

Sacks writes of another casualty of brain damage, in this case a man who suffered an injury to the head that, by damaging his olfactory tracts, robbed him entirely of his sense of smell. It was not a trivial loss: "Life lost a great deal of its savour," the man said. Recovery, he was told, was impossible. He was therefore both astonished and elated when his morning coffee and his pipe began to regain their flavor and aroma. He rushed to his doctor, who, after careful testing, told him that there had been in fact no recovery of the lost sense. Instead, it emerged, what had happened was that the man had developed "a greatly enhanced olfactory imagery, almost . . . a controlled hallucinosis." Thus, in situations "previously fraught with associations of smell," the man was able to "re-evoke" these smells with such intensity that he could believe them real. Even after learning that this was what was occurring, the man continued undaunted in the cultivation of these "smell-memories," so that the spring is for him truly fragrant.[23]

SURGERY WITH INADEQUATE ANESTHESIA, OR THE PAIN OF CHANGING ONE'S SELF-IMAGE

However adept one is at preserving one's memorabilia, a loss is still a loss. After losing some valued part of one's being, the person one was is no more. And one must adjust one's sense of oneself to take into account this unwanted change. There are a variety of ways that people can respond to the pain that comes from confronting a transformation of themselves from an accustomed and acceptable self to a new self that is hard to accept.

One response is anger. No wonder, say Levitt and Guralnick in *You Can Make It Back,* that those afflicted with illness often become enraged. Illness—"a ravager, a maker of skulls and ghosts"—can transform one so completely that, like Rip Van Winkle, one "awakens to an unfamiliar body," one sees in the mirror not "the faithful reflection, but the face of a stranger."[24] The reflection has broken faith; one has been betrayed. Hell hath no fury like one thus betrayed.

Another reaction is to avoid as much as possible the encounter with the "unfamiliar body." Betty Rollin describes the elaborate procedures by which, for a long time after her radical mastectomy, she avoided looking at the raw and scarred place on her body. The mirror is the enemy of those who cannot bear to see what they have become. In Robert Kavanaugh's *Facing Death,* there is a moving account written by a woman dying of cancer and being wasted not only by the disease but also by the abominable treatments by which cancer patients' lives are prolonged. "Every mirror in the house reflected only the tale of my indignity until Arnold took them all down."[25]

Even without illness, age itself performs plastic surgery on us, creating a new face whose wrinkles and sags and hollows are for many painful to behold. So distasteful did the French writer Valéry find his aging countenance that, he said, except to shave, he never looked at himself in the mirror. In his book *Learn to Grow Old,* Paul Tournier comments ruefully about this man "who cast his penetrating eye over the world, over mankind and over himself. And then, all at once, his glance is turned away—he cannot bear to look at his old age face to face."[26]

Of course, not every sign of distressing change can be avoided. Some changes force our attention upon them. Compelled to confront one's decline, one may be stricken with shame. It may not make rational sense to be ashamed of oneself for being disabled by some disaster. But rational logic does not always dictate psychologic. The philosopher John Rawls, for example, argues that no diminution of self-respect is warranted if something beyond one's control, such as illness, thwarts the fulfillment of one's "lifeplan." But Brody observes that, warranted or not, self-respect does suffer. To this I would add that if the positive aspects of one's self-image are bound up with capabilities that then disappear, then even if one does not blame oneself for the loss, how is one's self-image *not* going to be eroded?

It can be rewarding to identify with one's strongest, most capable part, but it is also dangerous—the pride that cometh before a fall. What happens if one outlives that special gift for which people have placed the laurels of honor upon one's head? Beisser, the young doctor-athlete struck down by polio, writes that "the athlete who insists he is a winner must deny his disabilities and defeats." This denial serves a temporary narcissistic purpose, but it places a trap along one's long-term path, for disability and defeat "are inevitable parts of the life cycle, as well as an athletic career." Later, when this "winner" must retire from his athletic career "because of age or injury, he feels like a loser, a role he has been taught to avoid like the plague."[27]

As suggested by the example of the athlete retiring because of age, even the successful completion of a Rawlsean life plan does not protect a person from having to deal eventually with the challenge to one's self-respect that comes from inevitable decline. Even after a life plan has been accomplished spectacularly and over a long span of time, a proud man like Igor Stravinsky describes his old age, with its various slips and "scatterbrained acts," as "a time of humiliations."[28]

In addition to the shame one may feel before one's own inner judging, there is shame before the eyes of others. Once again Moira Griffin shows a keen eye for those irrationalities in her own process that highlight the essential aspects of the struggle over the loss of the old identity. Visiting the neurologist for the first time in an effort to discover the source of the frightening changes taking place in her body, Griffin notices that she is working hard *not* to show the doctor the very symptoms she had come to present. "Though I'd wanted to see [the neurologist] so much, I was trying to hide my symptoms. It was a lot easier to talk about my odd problems than to *show* them—there was something shameful about my body being out of control."[29]

Just as one can avoid looking into the mirror, so can one avoid displaying before others one's damaged condition. In their book on old age, Erik Erikson and his coauthors describe a woman in her early nineties who, to spare herself the shame of moving falteringly in public, goes nowhere at all. "Although she might still attend the functions she has always enjoyed," say the authors, "she does not feel she could do so with the elegance she views as necessary to her image." "I'm not so much afraid of getting hurt," she says. "But what would it look like—a grown woman falling all over herself like a two-year-old."[30]

On the basis of pride of a kindred sort, Beethoven made a similar decision. "What a humiliation," he declared, to stand next to someone who could hear a distant flute while he heard nothing. "If I venture into the company of men, I am overcome by a burning terror, inasmuch as I fear to find myself in the danger of allowing my condition to be noticed." From such pride and such fear, Beethoven chose to "live like an outcast."[31]

It is touching to read, in the writings of one of Beethoven's disciples, Ludwig Rellstab, about a couple of incidents where Beethoven's disability was inadvertently made manifest, and about the mixture of pity and discretion with which the disciple, still holding his master in awe, responded. On the first occasion, he called Beethoven's attention to the sound of the shawm coming "bright and clear" through the woods. But Rellstab "observed from his expression that he did not hear the sounds," and it was then that Rellstab became convinced that Beethoven's hearing was impaired. Discreetly, "in order not to sadden him, I made believe that I too could not hear anything any more." On the second occasion, Beethoven was demonstrating a new piano to Rellstab, and with his eyes steadily upon the other man, Beethoven struck a chord, repeating it several times. "Never will another chord pierce me to the quick with such sadness and heartbreak. He has played C major in the right hand and B natural in the bass . . . and the greatest musician on earth could not hear the dissonance!"[32]

What a pity for a sensitivity so marvelous as Beethoven's hearing to be lost. But a proud man like Beethoven is not much comforted by pity. So the disciple bears these sad moments as private events, speaking of them only later, after his remarkable, angry, despairing, self-isolating master has perished.

When Aaron, my firstborn, was a baby, I recalled, I enjoyed referring to him by that hackneyed phrase "my pride and joy." (He was also "the crab-apple of my eye.") These days, it occurred to me, he is also my pride and, if not my humiliation, at least my embarrassment.

I had always known, of course, that someday Aaron would be stronger than I, but the acceleration of his ascent and of my decline brought the two lines to cross a good deal sooner than I had anticipated. The picture on the wall, taken two days after Nathaniel's birth, with me in the middle holding the infant in my hands and flanked on each side by Aaron and Terra, showed that it had not been so long since he barely came up to my shoulder. Now, I'm Shorty. I took great pleasure in seeing how Aaron had put on a good fifteen or twenty pounds of muscle in the past year or two. But it was hard to deal with my simultaneous loss of the same.

Now I turned to Aaron for my heavy lifting. For years, when I'd go to my mother's house she'd have a little list of things for me to do for her that she couldn't readily do for herself, like bring up the boxes with her winter clothes. Now I was caught—prematurely it seemed to me—in the downward turning of the generational cycle. As I built the stone walls to make my terraces on our steep hillside, there were some rocks that I'd leave for Aaron. It gratified him, I knew, to hear Natty say about some very heavy object, "We'll have to get Aaron to move that." I knew it would come, but this need to defer to my son in matters of strength seemed rather sudden and demoralizing. Having seen myself as still a young man just a few years earlier, suddenly I felt old and frail. I felt robbed and belittled.

How Aaron felt to see his father in decline he didn't say.

No Exit

Amid the frustration of just plain not feeling good and not being able to do anything about it, I have frequently wanted to shout: "I quit! I'm not going to sit still for this. I'm leaving!"

Over a decade ago, I recall, I was walking with my friend Alan Paskow in Rock Creek Park in Washington, D.C. We were discussing the very harrowing time I had recently gone through. My first marriage had crumbled. The manner of this relationship's dissolution was particularly wrenching, increasing to an unusually appalling level the rending of the flesh of one's life that ordinarily accompanies the end of an intimate relationship. Alan was commiserating with me about my tribulations, and I recounted to him a liberating discovery to which the experience had brought me. From the disintegration of the marriage, I had found a kind of bedrock of myself: whatever might happen in the circumstances of my life, I still had myself. With the realization that though everything could be taken from me, yet I would still retain what is essential, I emerged from that difficult transition stronger than before. My heart, though broken, was fortified.

Illness is different. If a relationship becomes sick, one can, however sadly, depart to make a new beginning. But what if the relationship is with one's own organism? As my words to April had suggested, the widow can remarry, but the deceased husband is stuck.

"If it were a horse I was riding that went lame or broke its neck," says R. S. of his aging body in Hans Zinsser's biography of him, "or a ship on which I was traveling that sprang a leak, I could transfer to another one and leave the old vehicle behind." But, "as it is, my mind and my spirit, my thoughts and my love, all that I really am, is inseparably tied up with the failing capacities of these outworn organs."[33] Inseparably tied. Some problems one simply cannot get away from.

R. S. is facing the fact that his "damaged body" will "extinguish me with it when it dies." For others, it is suffering itself from which one finds oneself inseparable. For them, death is not the problem but may seem the only conceivable solution. Beethoven gave serious thought to suicide. In *Darkness Visible,* William Styron's autobiographical memoir of his depressive illness, the author describes the night he spent on the brink of self-destruction. Suzy Szasz, worn down by the tortures of lupus, also gave thought to killing herself. The play in which Sartre presents his image of hell is called *No Exit;* for the sufferer from an illness to which no end is in sight, there seems to be no other way—save death—of quitting from an ongoing hell.

Even in the absence of great suffering, illness threatens the continuity of the old self. If one could only separate oneself off from the defect, the pain, the deterioration! If one could only preserve the sense that what is really essential remains intact.

An old woman in a wheelchair declares, "I'm very healthy; my leg is very sick."[34] Erikson and his coauthors present this as a healthy form of adaptation, and one can see why. No need here for a new identity. A line is drawn between the healthy and the sick, and the self—the sense of who the *I* is—stays securely on the right side of the line. Similarly, Joseph Heller, in his account of his siege under the onslaughts of Guillain-Barré syndrome, speaks as one whose central core went untouched, even as he was immobilized in bed for months, unable even to swallow: "*I* wasn't weak," he writes, "My *muscles were weak*."[35] There is loss here but, in some important sense, it is seen as peripheral.

Is this perspective—the maintenance of a sense of an underlying "I" who remains intact—one to which all who suffer loss can meaningfully aspire?

It is not one I have managed. I have been able to do it with pain. I have been able to do it with fatigue. But there has been a part of my own ordeal about which I have been unable say, "I have to deal with that problem, but the essential me remains unscathed." To the extent that the disability is entwined with one's consciousness, it seems to me, the "self" can no longer find sanctuary in some safe haven.

Consciousness is the king among our chess pieces. The other pieces play important roles, but they can be taken without stopping our game. When the opponent can take our king, it is checkmate.

The challenge of preserving one's identity in the midst of loss is, therefore, an important spiritual task, but it is not equally available to everyone. The old woman in the wheelchair has achieved something positive in being able to continue perceiving herself as basically healthy. But what could she do to maintain her identity if her affliction were Alzheimer's?

Recently, I delved into the aging experiences of a great many people. One discovery stands out for me: despite the evident willingness of many people to generalize from their own experience to proclaim about the nature of aging, the process of loss—and not just the reaction to loss—is really quite different for different people. Everyone ends up dying, but on the way some are robbed of mere trinkets while others have their riches snatched away.

Some preserve a fundamental sense that the self is intact, that aging does not violate the essence of one's identity; others feel they are living posthumously. Which people fall on which side of the line is determined *both* by differences in the kinds of losses they suffer and by differences in their ability to meet the spiritual challenge of suffering and loss.

Compare two statements, made in old age, by two luminaries of American cultural history. Henry Wadsworth Longfellow says: "In old age our bodies are worn-out instruments, on which the soul tries in vain to play the melodies of youth. But because the instrument has lost its strings, or is out of tune, it does not follow that the musician has lost his skill."[36] For Longfellow, evidently, there is a sense of an unchanging musician who abides independently of the deterioration of the instrument. But then consider, by contrast, the lament of the noted art historian Bernard Berenson: "I have lost my grip in almost every way. . . . [The loss of intellectual powers makes me] feel ever so diminished, so superfluous, so unworthy of all the alarming expenses and trouble to others of keeping me alive. . . . I gasp and yearn and fall back humiliated."[37] It may not be irrelevant that, when he penned these words, Berenson was nearly twenty years older than Longfellow was when he died: had Longfellow also lived into his nineties, would he have continued to speak of a musician persisting with undiminished skill? On the other hand, in Berenson's humiliation at being unable to "recall the reasoning by which I arrived at my convictions," does not Berenson disclose himself to be ensnared in the grip of a narcissistic identification with a particular ability to perform?

But, narcissism aside, it seems to me that there is no way the "self" can escape the darkening of the mind. I cannot see how one with Alzheimer's might say, "I am perfectly healthy; it's my mind that is disappearing."

The Slow Disappearance of Ray Doernberg is the subtitle of Myrna Doernberg's book about her husband's decline and death from another form of dementia (Binswanger's disease). In one scene of this story, the wife wanted to say to a group of people assembled to help deal with the progressive incompetence of this man, "You should have known him before. You would not believe what has happened to this man."[38] Unlike with the still skillful Longfellow, or even the humiliated Berenson, it is not Ray Doernberg but his wife who writes the testimony about his loss.

As with the extinguishing of the light through dementia, so with the darkness of depression. What is the meaning of Virginia Ironside's statement, "It cannot be said too strongly that a depressed person and his or her depression are separate"?[39] We live, inescapably, through our consciousness. One might learn to ignore and rise above the pain in one's foot, or to take quiet pleasure in contemplating the shifting play of sunlight in the clouds, when illness or age has depleted the energy that once allowed more rambunctious delights. But when the capacity for delight is itself maimed, when the very color of one's experience is itself tinged with an unspeakable darkness, what recourse is there then?

In Styron's well-known book about his own depression, he describes how his surroundings took on a darker tone: "The shadows of nightfall seemed more somber, my mornings were less buoyant, walks in the woods became less zestful."[40] Styron describes his feelings on a trip to Paris to accept a prize for his writing. Instead of being able to take the pleasure he should be having, Styron reports, in a passage reminiscent to me of my feeling about the people coming to visit the author of *The Parable of the Tribes,* finding himself "engulfed by a toxic and unnameable tide that obliterated any enjoyable response to the living world." How does one spiritually transcend a toxic cloud that is lodged in one's very spirit?

Ironside's statement about the separation between the disease of depression and its victim may make sense if it means that depression can end, that it can be successfully treated, that the person who once was can be resurrected. The depression and the sufferer are proven separable once the latter continues without the former. Styron's own account is proof that one might outlive one's living death. But while the toxic cloud is there, was Styron separable from his depression?

As one who has observed his own emotional life carefully for many years, I have been convinced that my own malady is not to be explained in terms of what I understand depression to be. That is, it is clear that the coming and going of the cloud has in no way been governed by the ups and downs of my emotional state. Yet, whatever the source of the cloud, the effect has certainly been depressive: the lack of luster, the suppressed capacity for response, an impoverishment even of my dream life. And it has been this depressive aspect that has been the loss most difficult for me to accept. Injury to the part of me through which I had made contact with the sacred realm is the injury hardest to bear.

André Gide labels as an illusion the idea that "the last years of life can be devoted to a more energetic search for God." He is, of course, generalizing from his own experience of aging, which is one in which there is a "progressive blunting of the senses, a sort of stupor numbs one's being; and, as the outside world loses its lustre and its incentives, one's vigor fails." But Gide captures in a marvelous image his sense of a fundamental loss of one's essence that takes place as "a certain dreary indifference takes possession of the spirit, already pruned like those trees which the woodcutter has prepared for felling."[41]

NO GREAT TALENT

"I'm not sure I can take this indefinitely," I had said to my brother on the phone. Now, coming down the hill from the mailbox, Ed's letter in hand, I was touched by his concern. I didn't think I was signaling any suicidal intention, but Ed was not taking any chances. He wanted to make sure he knew just what I meant.

So what *was* I saying? That I don't know how to quit and I can't stand this continual defeat. It was no coincidence that my call to Ed came just after I'd tried a new approach that had seemed so hopeful, but which had collapsed and brought me back—for the umpteenth time—to square one. I called Ed to tell him, no, I wasn't signaling a self-destructive impulse. It was more that I was insisting that there has got to be some way of throwing in the towel, of accepting defeat. But I didn't know how to throw in the towel in a match where the bell never rings. My moment-to-moment experience makes me feel like a loser: I didn't like that feeling, and I hadn't found any way around it.

"So, boychick," my brother asked, "what is it that makes losing such a big deal?"

Our conversation went on to explore how important it had always been to me to play to win. We ended on the note: maybe, if I can't win against this malady-that-lingers-on, I can grow past the narcissistic component in my response to losing to it. Take the insult out of the injury.

That night, lying in bed, I mused about how life certainly does not always deal to one's long suit. Wouldn't you know I'd have to wrestle with loss. As a kid, I recall, I had difficulty accepting a loss so mundane as the replacing of our old sofa. (I did not want members of our family talking disparagingly of the sofa within earshot of it, lest we hurt the feelings of something on which we had spent so many cozy hours.) When the first car to which I ever felt attached—a 1946 Nash named Sampson—died a natural death, I protested its being carted off to the junkyard. We should, I maintained, bury it in our yard. Now I thought of that old joke: How many Virginians does it take to change a lightbulb? Four, one to change the bulb and three to talk about how great the old bulb was. Now I had become a Virginian, and while that seemed strange—what am I doing in the heart of the Confederacy?—it was at least fitting that, like the Virginian in the joke, I'm mourning the dimming of the old bulb.

It was clear I had no great talent for dealing with loss.

As I thought about it, I could see how I came by my lack of this particular talent. The greatest determinant of the emotional climate in which I grew up was my mother—not only because she was, like most mothers of her generation, far more often with us children than was our father (off for long hours at the office), but also because she is a powerful presence. She was, for my brother and me, a marvelous storyteller who made the people and places of her own early life as vivid for us as our own immediate surroundings. And prominent in the emotional space opened by the link between her imagination and ours was the theme of loss still being grieved.

Mom's father died when she was not yet four, leaving a void with respect to both love and security that was never to be filled. This tragic story of young love and early death is now the heart of my mother's major piece of writing—a just-written novel based on her mother's life. And I in turn was brought up on stories of this woman—larger than life in her wisdom and charm—who died of a failing heart when my mother, in her twenties, was soon to be married. Then after a quarter-century of a successful marriage, Mom lost my father to cancer. In the decades since then, my mother continued to live a vital and creative life; she also still wrote more of her poetry about grief than about any other subject.

The fact that loss is a part of life is something I had known in some way from the beginning. But how one could come to terms with that loss, how one could let go and make some kind of new beginning, I would have to figure out for myself.

It is true that life does not always deal to one's long suit. But then it came to me why just the opposite would be true: whatever one can deal with gets dealt with, and then one goes on to the next thing; what one cannot deal with, however, stays stuck in one's hand until one does deal with it. It is the problem one is ill-equipped for that will not go away, and so looms larger in one's experience.

Perhaps nothing in this whole struggle seemed to me so deadening as the feeling of being *stuck:* not just in a place I didn't want to be, but getting nowhere. Again and again, I would feel that I was back at square one, in the same predicament, feeling the same frustrations. Perhaps it was not the *situation* so much that had me stuck as my *response* to it. Movement is the essence of the animate; perhaps it was my inability to move on that was the essence of my living posthumously.

CHAPTER 3

Struck by the Obvious

What Does It Mean to Know That One Is Mortal?

On a snowy morning one January, Terra came to me and said, "Daddy, I can't find Jason anywhere." Jason was our cat, at seventeen years old about a decade older than his human sister, Terra. Before I had children, I had often referred to Jason as my firstborn son. I had named him Jason after my father, Jacob, who had died a couple of years before Jason was born.

I had adopted Jason and his sister, Juliet, together when they were seven weeks old. Juliet never made it to maturity, because one night on the Oakland, California, corner where we lived she was caught by a pack of dogs. I got to her quickly—she still had enough strength that in her panic, when I picked her up, she could bite through my thumbnail—but she did not make it to the vet. Over the next week, I learned that a cat can mourn. Jason, who had always slept curled with his sister like a yang with a yin, eventually stopped looking for his sister and went on with life a bit more solemn than he'd been before.

Around that time, my ladylove of that era of my life, Marilyn, moved in with me, along with her black cat, Sheba. Jason quickly taught the skittish Sheba that having another cat for a friend could be a beautiful thing, and the two of them became buddies, chasing each other around the house when it was hunting time, licking each other clean when it was time to settle down. But after about half a year, Sheba caught feline leukemia, and we had to take her to the vet to be euphemized. This time, Jason's mourning was even deeper. It was well over a month before he ceased to grieve, and when he emerged from it it seemed to me there was something very deep and very serious in his view of things. He was a year old at that point, and his manner told you that he understood that life is not just a frivolous game.

Marilyn and I had two very sweet years together in California and then Connecticut, but we were not destined for the long haul, and so I found myself alone—or rather, it was just Jason and me. Jason and I went on to live together in the mountains and then the desert of Arizona, then in rural and then suburban Maryland. My first marriage began, Aaron and Terra were born, and the marriage ended dismayingly. Jason was still there. *The Parable of the Tribes* was finally published. April and I met and then lived in the house by Sligo Creek, and Jason was still my companion.

Jason was the most noble animal I had ever known: always dependable and considerate, always a good uncle to the kittens that sometimes came into our family, always trusting that whatever indignities I subjected him to—such as catheterization for urinary blockages—were for his sake and should therefore be accepted in a cooperative spirit, always solid in his judgment—the kind of fellow you would want for your attorney if you were going to have a cat for a lawyer.

But Jason had grown old. He was practically blind now, and he walked unsteadily. He still relished going outside—to the extent that he could still relish anything—and I wasn't about to deny the cat that had roamed forests of ponderosa pine and fields of growing corn such pleasures as he could still get from nighttimes by Sligo Creek. But I could tell from the expression on his face that life was no longer a pleasure for him. He was failing.

When Terra came to me, wondering where Jason was, I got up quickly and dressed, with a feeling of foreboding. The new snow had melted on our street, but was still a couple of inches deep everywhere else. I called for Jason, and looked for his footprints. Then I tried the hypothesis I hoped I would not confirm, looking for gray fur by the side of the road. Up one side, then down the other until Terra and I approached the bridge crossing the creek. There, about five feet from the road, on a mound of snow a bit behind the concrete abutment of the bridge, I found him. He was dead.

"Oh, Jason. Oh, Jason," I kept saying gently to this forlorn and stiff furry object he had become. Then the tears and sobs came. Never in my life had I cried so freely. It just flowed. I turned to Terra to deal with her visible distress, holding her to me, her seven-year-old's tresses against my winter coat. "We're going to have to say good-bye to our friend, Jason," I told her. Then, looking at her, I grasped that it was less Jason's cold corpse that was upsetting her than the equally unfamiliar sight of her father in tears.

To Terra, I could see, I was supposed to be the steady and un-flappable one. I was the one who had comforted her, the soft-hearted daughter condemned to watch her parents break apart, while she cried her eyes out over the scene in *Dumbo* when the little elephant is separated from his mother. I was the one who had run home with her a half-year earlier when the Takoma Park fireworks bursting over our heads, evoking "oohs" and "ahs" from the crowd, threw her into an unconquerable panic. I was supposed to be the rock on which she could found her security.

"I'm okay, Terra," I reassured her. "You remember the song? 'Crying gets the sad out.' It's part of saying good-bye to someone I love, who's gone now. Jason is gone. This is just what is left when the cat we love stopped being."

"Why did he die?"

"He was old, sweetie. He had a long and full life. It was a good life, but it was coming to an end. My guess is that, bad as his vision was, he accidentally wandered in front of a car. Life wasn't much fun for Jason, anymore. So this is probably as good an end to his life as he could have gotten. . . . Come, let's get Aaron and bury Jason in our yard."

So we did. Each of us stood over the piece of earth I'd dug up and then covered over Jason, and said a few words of appreciation and farewell.

Later that evening, Terra stood in front of me. "Daddy, are we ever going to see Jason again?"

"No, we won't. Dying is forever."

She took that in for a minute. "Daddy, are you going to die?"

SMALL CONSOLATION

It was interesting how my illness had changed the way it felt for me to think about my mortality. It was not only in the fairly obvious way, that feeling lousy suggested that one might feel worse, that losing vitality presaged losing life. Beyond that, the fact of my inevitable mortality had, quite ironically, provided me a way of coming to terms with my illness.

As I sat in the orchard, working on this book, another of my favorite Woody Allen lines served to console. "When Mozart was my age," the line goes, "he had been dead for seven years." Why was this consoling? It was one of those "I met a man who had no feet" things: how could I feel too sorry for myself for having no shoes? And if it's *Mozart* who has no feet, who am I to feel so terribly cheated to lose some years of my prime when Mozart, at my age, was already dead? Contemplating the mortality of others who have gone before me and whom I hold in the highest respect, and relating my decline to their fate, helped me simultaneously to come to terms with what had happened to me and to acknowledge more deeply that I, too, will die.

And there was another way it has worked.

I could see now that a major contributor to my anguish was that, by virtue of my tacit assumptions, my loss seemed infinite. The idea that "Maybe I'll *never* feel any better" is particularly bitter if one assumes that, if it weren't for this problem, I would *always* feel better—that is, for time without end. If at some level I believed myself immortal, to be sick and not get better is to be Prometheus tied to a rock for eternity. This disclosed how, at some level, I have been living in an "eternal now." Time had never stopped yet, for me, so why should it ever? Any loss of vitality that did not end therefore appeared infinite. Coming to terms with so great a loss is hard to do.

Accepting my mortality thus greatly reduced my loss. "I'd have lost it eventually anyway" actually was consoling. Like the time I was so bitterly disappointed as a kid when the flu kept me from going to a much-awaited Detroit Tigers game: it turned out the game was canceled because of rain anyway, which made not seeing a game so much easier to bear. Still no game, but so much easier to accept when I knew that in any case I wouldn't have gotten all those goodies.

In these ways, in my search for solace for my more immediate loss, I was led to embrace my eventual mortality. But the kicker was this: really looking at the fact that I will die was no small thing.

I KNEW IT ALL ALONG

I have a clear recollection of thinking, on the morning of my seventh birthday, that I was now one-tenth of the way to a person's allotted three score and ten. And one-tenth seemed alarmingly larger than infinitesimal. I was big on numbers then, and I calculated the number of days in an average human life. Coming up with a number roughly equivalent to the population of my then hometown, East Lansing, Michigan, I figured that in such a town an average of one person should die each day. I knew that one day, inevitably, it would be my turn.

Admittedly, I wasn't entirely convinced. For one thing, in the early 1950s there was in America a buoyant faith that the leaps and bounds of technological progress would rapidly overtake the limits to which human life had been subject. This cultural atmosphere encouraged me in the hope, perhaps even the expectation, that by the time I was old enough to worry about aging, the process of aging might well have been abolished. Aside from these hopes for technological salvation, I had one other basis for believing I might escape what seemed to be the common destiny of humankind: an underlying (and until now secret) belief that I was somehow special. I have since come to understand that it is not readily apparent to other people that I of all people should be immune to the adversities of human life, so I will not endeavor here to persuade anyone of the reasonableness of that belief. When I was a child, however, it was possible for me to entertain a small hope that the Angel of Death would pass me over indefinitely.

But, aside from such lingering hopes, I also knew that time had me in its inexorable grasp, that though I was a boy I would become a man, that though now a child I would have children, that I would be pulled on beyond the prime of life into a time of decline. I knew that the passage of time would inescapably bring me to death, that the world had once existed before me and that it would later continue on without me.

I *knew* all that, yet now, when life has placed such facts right in front of me, that I might see them more clearly, I meet them with great surprise. How can it be that one can discover with astonishment something one has long known?

STRUCK BY THE OBVIOUS

This matter of my mortality is not the first thing I have known and not known at the same time. Surprises that are also not surprises happen to me all the time.

Sitting in my living room watching the news on television, I see a reporter talking into the microphone in some frigid outdoor location. With every breath, a cloud of steam becomes momentarily visible, and I feel a momentary shock to discover that this reporter is a creature who breathes, like I do, pulling air into and out of the body, infusing it with warmth and moisture.

When I talk to groups about the marvelous and terrible story of our species, I often try to evoke that we are creatures embedded in the vast panorama of life on Earth. I look around the auditorium, at these faces connected to bodies mostly covered by clothing, and say: "Right now, inside each one of us, within a bony rib cage, a heart is beating, pumping a fluid to bathe each cell, a fluid that has the same salt content as the ancient seas where our one-celled ancestors first arose." I am hoping my words will help my listeners experience more deeply their connection with the whole history of life on this planet. I can't always tell how effective my words are on the audience, but not infrequently I myself will feel a sense of amazement—not necessarily because of the mind-boggling stream of time that has brought us to that moment, but simply to be aware that each body in the room contains a beating heart.

I came of age in the 1950s, a time when as many as possible of the traces of human sexuality were covered up. Yet there we children were, undeniable traces of what our parents had been up to. My friends and I both knew and had difficulty believing what the evidence clearly showed about that whole parental generation. And when, as I grew up and even after I grew up, I had occasion to discover that some women indeed possessed those parts of the body that our society generally insists on keeping covered, that discovery was always accompanied by some astonishment.

There are over five billion people in the world, each one an "I" to him- or herself, each one with concerns and struggles and feelings as important to him or her as mine are to me. I know this, but at times it will hit me with considerable force as an astounding realization. That person waiting for a bus is living a life, just as I am; or, driving in some strange and out of the way place, I'll be startled to realize about some house tucked away on a bend in the road, this place is home for someone, the place where they wake up every morning. The notion that, in the words of the old television series, "There are eight million stories in the Naked City" is a powerful one, no less so, apparently, for being "obvious."

EXTRA! EXTRA! READ ALL ABOUT IT

To write this book, I have had to deal with various fears of possible embarrassment. At the heart of this exploration are certain realizations, many of them of quite obvious: that I live in this body, that this body was assembled at a particular time, and that it will, in the fullness of time, be correspondingly disassembled; that my position in the great scheme of things is fundamentally the same as everyone else's, which is rather piddling. As I contemplate sharing these profundities, an image of readers' lips curled with scorn makes me timorous: "This is news?" I imagine my readers asking derisively. I can see the headlines now—"Author Discovers Death"—while the story goes on with the news flash that a "theorist of the evolution of civilization brings another stunning discovery: 'All men are mortal,' Schmookler claims, 'and that includes me.' " At some especially unsure moments, I wonder if I'm the only one who finds these matters difficult to grasp. Maybe other people—perhaps not as narcissistic as I am, or more firmly rooted in their bodies than I—don't have to wrestle with these matters. Maybe even on this page I am making a fool of myself.

As part of the research for this book, and as a precaution against such embarrassment, I did an informal survey among my friends, especially those with the insight and expertise to work with people at a deep psychological level. Is it just some weirdness of mine, I wanted to know, that makes these questions seem important? The responses I got were reassuring. I may be weird, I was told, but that kind of weirdness is something I have in common with other people. ("We want a second opinion that says, Don't worry, you are going to live forever."[1])

Apparently, there are some important, and rather obvious, things that most of us, at least, have trouble getting through our heads. Truths at once obvious and surprising. We know them, but we also don't know them. Which raises the question: what does it mean to *know* something?

COMING TO UNDERSTAND

In our society, the predominant notion of knowledge is superficial "quiz show" knowledge. Either you know it or you don't. Who was the president before Lincoln? What is the capital of Kansas? We honor the master of such trivial pursuits. In our institutions of higher learning, successful initiates—those awarded the Ph.D.—are those who contribute "new" knowledge, however inconsequential, believing as we do that the amassing of increments of knowledge of this sort amounts to the progress of human understanding.

This is the culture—both the larger society with its quiz shows, and the smaller culture of academia—into which I was socialized.

And consequently, I feel a good deal more secure taking the floor to give voice to something other people don't know—even in the quiz show sense—than to explore something everyone knows— something like that first premise of the prototypical syllogism, "All men are mortal (and women too)." But the more I have devoted myself to trying to discover, and to articulate, what is important for a person to know, the more inadequate quiz show knowledge—or even scientific knowledge—seems to be. And the more I am impressed that the central philosophical challenge facing human beings is to *really know* some truths that most of us know only superficially.

The answer to the question "Do I know I am mortal?" is a good deal more complex than "yes" or "no" because a human being is a complex entity. On most matters of any importance, we are of more than one mind. And these minds can diverge in interesting ways. One central issue, then, is how well we have *integrated* one bit of knowledge with everything else we know or believe or feel.

This is certainly true of absorbing some great loss we have suffered, but the challenge of integrating our knowledge is hardly confined to that realm.

In part, the challenge can be seen as a cognitive one. When some new and important bit of knowledge comes in, what happens to all those other notions we thought we had believed that now stand in need of revision? I find that old images die rather hard under the impact of new and contradicting images. Often, after a momentary jolt from an unexpected discovery, my mind will revert to its old habits of thought.

When I was twelve or so, my father took me one evening to hear the astronomer Harlow Shapley speak at the University of Minnesota. Using slides and other visual aids, Shapley showed us the immensity of the universe: distances measured in the millions and billions of light-years (when light can travel almost from here to the moon in a single second), the cosmos speckled with count-less galaxies (when each galaxy is huge beyond comprehensibility). It blew my mind. For a few hours, I really did feel I lived on a speck of dust. The vastness of this perspective was unsettling, so difficult was it to integrate into my normal mundane frame of reference. For a short while, I walked around with new eyes. But soon my world resumed its familiar, manageable form. Now, there are moments when the astronomical perspective will hit me like a revelation, and then I really *know* that this world which is so vast to me is but the tiniest grain. Most of the time, however, I live in a pre-Copernican world that I "know" to be an illusion.

A more recent example arose about a year ago when I read a manuscript by a colleague of mine, John Mack of Harvard University. Mack had undertaken a psychological study of a number of people who report themselves to have been abducted by creatures not from Earth. What emerged surprised me. I had expected the data to show these reports to be symptomatic of psychoses or other delusional conditions. But that is not what I found. In light of the marked similarities among quite independent descriptions by separate individuals, I felt compelled to consider seriously the possibility that these strange reports are valid. If these reports are true, however, large chunks of my worldview stand in need of revision: a world being visited by other sentient beings, with advanced powers and a special interest in the fate of this planet and in us as a species, is very different from the world in which I have believed myself to be living. I don't change my image of the world very readily, however. My reaction, I observed, was to enter into a somewhat agitated and heightened state of awareness for a few days, and then gradually to relinquish the new, discrepant element and revert back to the world as I had known it before.

It is as though a trail was opened up in my mind, but then, in the absence of further wanderings along it propelled by new data, the trail becomes overgrown again with the vegetation of my habitual beliefs. Should some aliens appear on prime-time television making an announcement of their intentions, I expect the residual traces of the trail Mack forged would enable me to understand the import of their landing and to adjust to it more quickly than I would have if I had never read Mack's unsettling work. But I expect even then I'd be much like those cold warriors who could not believe Gorbachev was truly a different kind of Soviet leader until the Soviet Union had virtually dissolved.

Likewise, sometimes the trail blazed in my mind years ago by Harlow Shapley directs what I perceive when I look into the night sky from my Shenandoah Valley ridge. "Shenandoah" is said to come from a Native American word meaning "daughter of the stars," and on some Shenandoah nights the number of stars visible is quite overwhelming. Once in a while, from my deck at night, I can recapture the sense of mind-boggling vastness that Shapley's lecture first opened up. For the most part, however, I stay fixed in my more domesticated geocentric room of which even the Shenandoah sky is just a nifty ceiling.

New paths do not readily displace those that are well-worn in our minds. In his well-known book *The Structure of Scientific Revolutions,* Thomas Kuhn suggests that the way a new scientific paradigm replaces an old one is not by the persuasion of the adherents of the old to adopt the new so much as by the holders of the old belief dying out and being replaced by younger people brought up on the new system of understanding. It is not the changing of minds, in other words, so much as the turnover in the cast of characters. Old habits of thought are hard for us to change, even in the face of new knowledge.

If that resistance to change is so strong even in a realm as purely cerebral as scientific theory, imagine how much more so it must be in those areas of our beliefs and habits whose tendrils delve below rational cognition into the very fiber of our lives and feelings.

My mother tells me that every time she climbs the stairs and finds herself laboring, finds herself lacking the energy of her youth, she is surprised. She knows she's not young anymore—not under thirty-nine years old anyway—but the signs of it are still unexpected.

The death of a loved one is a still more dramatic example. Such a loss is something we can simultaneously know and most emphatically persist in not knowing. Part of this is because the relationship is so entwined into the trellis of our lives that we cannot quickly grasp the void left by the death. The power of the knowledge is so great that the grief from the loss may darken every waking moment. Yet at the same time, a newly widowed woman may continue setting the table for two. As other examples of "continuing the habits of the relationship," Judy Tatelbaum in *The Courage to Grieve* cites "buying the deceased's favorite food, making an appointment for the deceased, or automatically including the deceased in some social engagement."[2] Integrating the new knowledge of loss into one's moment-by-moment management of life takes time when the person lost was part of the very foundation of one's life.

When a parent dies—even the parent of an adult—there is a special difficulty in reconfiguring one's world, for the parent had *always* been there before. There was no time before one met one's parents; they always loomed large over the entire landscape. Suddenly, something seemingly as permanent as a mountain is removed. In her book *After Great Pain,* Diane Cole, in describing her difficulty in accepting her mother's death, tells how when the phone would ring, she would "run to pick it up. Mom had always found a way to call. . . . Irrationally, and yet yearningly, I wondered, could it be her now?"[3]

The $64,000 question is not at the quiz show level of "Can you tell us, Diane, is your mother alive or dead?" It is, rather, "Have you been able to integrate your knowledge of her death into a new sense of yourself and your life in the world?"

SAY IT AIN'T SO, JOE

There is a crucial, additional reason why it is difficult really to know that death comes for us all, that those we love and we ourselves will all return to dust. That reason is that this particular knowledge is not only powerfully disruptive of the world as we have known it; it is also quite painful. In proportion to that pain, we are motivated to protect ourselves from full knowledge.

If the technological breakthrough I anticipated as a child finally made death optional, we would doubtless have some difficulty adjusting. I can imagine hearing the startling news that there is now readily available a potion that, when drunk, makes one immune to death for a year, and then sitting down to pay the annual premium on my life insurance policy. But though even welcome news can be hard to integrate, the difficulty is greatly compounded when the truth is one we wish with all our hearts were not true.

While we are in our prime, we would like to believe we will enjoy our powers forever. Professional football players still in their playing years, according to psychologist Tony Bober, tend to practice denial. "It isn't going to end," they think. "I'm not going to end up with some disability."[4] Of course it will end, and for a high proportion of them, their rough sport will leave them some disabling injury to remember it by.

People in our society may have a special difficulty dealing with getting to the far side of life's hill. Compared with the values in most traditional societies, our society holds in contempt the characteristics that come with aging. It is youth's vigor and pristine looks we idealize.

A few years back, the creators of a new television series had the bad marketing judgment to call their program "Middle Ages." This would-be prime-time look at post-prime life was well-received by the critics, but "viewers never gave it a chance." "The name was a colossal mistake," said producer Stan Rogow. " 'Middle age' is this horrible-sounding thing you've heard throughout your life and hated." As the low ratings for the show became evident, Rogow said to himself, "We have a problem here, and it's called denial."[5]

Some of the elderly among us, determined to deny their descent through the aging process, are ripe for caricature. Malcolm Muggeridge, elderly himself, found occasion to do some picking. In a withering description of life among the geriatric set in a Florida retirement community, Muggeridge describes how "everything was done to make us feel that we were not really aged, but still full of youthful zest and expectations." Through his eyes, the results of the efforts at denial appear grotesque: "Withered bodies arrayed in dazzling summer-wear, hollow eyes glaring out of garish caps, skulls plastered with cosmetics, lean shanks tanned a rich brown, bony buttocks encased in scarlet trousers."[6]

Is aging really inherently so ugly, with its withered bodies and bony buttocks, I wonder, or is this perception an artifact of our cultural taste? There is little in the world I find more beautiful than an ancient tree, with its gnarly limbs, its deep-wrinkled bark, its cavernous holes where owls might dwell. Might one reasonably see in a human body, likewise close to its return to the earth, a similar beauty? In twentieth-century America, in any event, these are not our standards of beauty.

Thus it is that as members of my generation move through the midpoint of the demographic python, there has been an "increase in a once rare condition called dysmorphophobia—the intense but unfounded fear of looking ugly."[7] Thus have my researches disclosed how my own weirdness—my being taken aback to discover that, like Socrates in the syllogism, I will prove mortal—is not so idiosyncratic. My brother, Ed, recently sent me a *Newsweek* cover story about the baby boomers approaching the discovery, as the caption on the cover put it, "Oh God . . . I'm really turning 50!" Ed's point was the cosmic coincidence that this issue hit the news-

stands on December 5, 1992—his fiftieth birthday! (Since I am on
the snout of the pig in the python, an avant-garde baby boomer
born in April 1946, the appearance of that issue of *Newsweek* on my
fiftieth birthday might have been expected. But I'll admit that its
showing up on my brother's fiftieth [1942–   ] does seem rather
cosmic.) But the story was also useful for my work on this book. In
it, a California psychiatrist, Harold Bloomfield, says of the baby
boomers, "This group was somehow programmed to never get
older."[8] When reality comes into conflict with programmed expectations, the result is a difficulty in integrating the news. Oh God
. . . can it be true?

Where does such "programming" come from? Perhaps it comes
from an unrealistic "happy-face" view of life that is another part of
our cultural outlook. The terms of our relationship to life, some
suggest, have become unbalanced, preparing us for grabbing all the
gusto we can get, but not for the pain and hardship. Married to life
for better but not for worse.

The confrontation with death is inevitably painful, but all the
more difficult when our orientation toward life fails to include such
a basic and inescapable aspect of our existence. This difficulty can
breed various rituals of denial. There is, for example, the wide-
spread practice of lying to the dying patient about "the gravity of
his condition." Though this practice emerged fairly recently in
historical terms, there has already been time, according to Philippe
Ariès, for its motivational basis to change. It began, Ariès says in his
Western Attitudes Toward Death, as an effort on the part of the
healthy "to spare the sick person, to assume the burden of ordeal."
But what was originally done out of consideration for the afflicted
soon became part of a strategy for self-protection for the healthy.
Programmed by modern culture to believe as a "given that life is
always happy or should always seem to be so," the healthy now lie
to the sick, "no longer for the sake of the dying person" but to

spare themselves "the disturbance and the overly strong and un-bearable emotion cased by the ugliness of dying and by the very presence of death in the midst of a happy life."[9]

Unable to gaze upon the ugly face of death, the healthy and the living labor to obscure the realities of dying and the dead. Barney G. Glaser and Anselm L. Strauss describe how nurses can conspire in the denial of the true condition of the terminal patient. "We remember one elaborate pretense ritual involving a husband and wife who had won the nurses' sympathy. The husband simply would not recognize that his already comatose wife was approach-ing death, so each morning the nurses carefully prepared her for his visit, dressing her for the occasion and making certain that she looked as beautiful as possible."[10] No amount of cosmetics, of course, can obscure the fact of death once it occurs, but the effort to evade reality can continue nonetheless. It is for such evasion and denial that modern funeral customs are frequently criticized. Vivian Rakoff, for example, writes that the American funeral ritual "is constructed in such a way as to deny all its most obvious implica-tions."[11] And Zachary Heller says of these customs that the "cos-metics, elaborate pillowed and satined coffins, and green artificial carpeting that shields the mourners from seeing the raw earth of the grave are all ways in which the culture enables us to avoid confronting the reality of death."[12] On the basis of their experi-ence as funeral directors in contemporary America, Ron and Jane Nichols observe that "the acceptance of death and the resulting ability to move through the grief work is severely inhibited by the notion that death cannot possibly be part of the American dream and the Good Life."[13]

A failure to make provision in one's view of life for the inevitable will, of course, inevitably lead to problems.

Denial can work well in the short run. Living in a world without death can be felicitous—until one must actually deal with death. I think of the joke about a man who fell off the top of a 100-story building; asked how he was doing as he passed the fiftieth floor, he said, "So far, so good." That's the sense in which much of our denial of death "works." The Nicholses go on to tell about their own experience of being present to the death of their father. Having observed the impediments to the work of grief from people's "tendency . . . to withdraw from the death experience and to seek a functionary to perform the whole task," their personal experience "revealed to us the benefits of moving closer to the death experience."[14] They were able to achieve a kind of emotional completion.

THE NEW DIRTY SECRET

Professionals in the field of psychotherapy are virtually unanimous in affirming the importance of the grieving process. Yet Ariès observed that—as of a couple of decades ago, in any event—the mainstream culture had quite assiduously ignored such psychological counsel, persisting in the "dangerous and absurd" ethic that suppresses mourning. This contrasts, Ariès points out, with the culture's popularization and assimilation of the psychologists' insights into sexuality and child development. Ariès interprets resistance so strong as a sign of the "force of the feeling that drives people to exclude death."[15]

Death and sexuality, paired here in Ariès's analysis, recur together as a striking motif in the modern literature on death. The Catholic priest Robert Kavanaugh describes the reaction of friends—"they gulp and look away"—when he tells them he is writing a book about death. "I feel like the teller of bawdy jokes in a girl scout camp or convent parlor."[16] The English anthropologist Geoffrey Gorer seems to have helped forge that link, writing in the 1950s about the "pornography of death." The similarity is noted between the shame surrounding sexuality in Victorian times and a similar discomfort regarding death in our times. "In the twentieth century . . . there seems to have been an unremarked shift in prudery; whereas copulation has become more and more 'mentionable,' particularly in Anglo-Saxon societies, death has become more and more 'unmentionable' *as a natural process.*"[17] And Malcolm Muggeridge notes that "death becomes the dirty little secret that sex once was."[18]

As in the case of Victorian sexual repression, an essential dimension of human experience is relegated to the shadows. Just as sexuality is made dirty by shame, and finds furtive expression in a variety of less healthy forms, so does the shame surrounding death and mourning work to abort the healthy work of grief. Studies clearly show how important emotional support from others is in the mourning process, yet, as Ariès noted in his earlier book about death, modern society has developed an ethic in which "one has the right to cry only if no one else can see or hear." And then comes again that intriguing linkage connecting the shame attached to the process by which life is begun and that attached to life's end. "Solitary and shameful mourning is the only recourse, like a sort of masturbation."[19]

In the past two decades, the shroud of secrecy surrounding death and its accompanying emotions has begun to lift. The hospice movement, among others, has brought some humanity back into the process of dying, helping both the dying and their families experience that event as a meaningful part of life. Death and bereavement have become recognized fields for scientific study and therapeutic work. Some healing, in other words, may be under way.

Death remains, however, a pariah among us, at once stalking our society and relegated to the shadows, both well known to us and kept a stranger.

THE GREATEST TEACHER

To know something intellectually is easy. To have that knowledge permeate one's being can be very hard.

It took me a while to figure out that logical argument alone does not govern what beliefs people will hold and which they will reject. My early belief in the power of argument grew out of the process of disputation with my father, an academic economist. Growing up with my father, one had to be prepared to defend what one had to say—not against hostile attack but against tests and challenges. If I met his opposing arguments successfully, I could change his thinking on the point at issue. A belief, with him, was like the king in a chess game: if he had no moves left to rescue it, he would recognize that he was checkmated and that the game was over.

Some implicit belief that all readers would be like my father governed, I believe, the way I wrote *The Parable of the Tribes*. At the beginning of my career as a writer, I crafted argument, trying to make it so irresistible that the reader had no choice by the end but to knock over the king of his former understanding and capitulate to my theory. My writing there was invariably directly engaged with the immediate point at issue, as I drove the reader inescapably toward our destination, like a cowboy driving a herd down a canyon along a western arroyo.

My experience with readers has taught me a few things since then. Over the years, a few readers of my first book have actually told me, "I resisted you for the first half of the book, but eventually I saw that you had closed off all the escape routes and I had to admit, reluctantly, that you were right." But these are rare birds. More typically, I have discovered, one can "win" an argument and the other person doesn't even notice! Checkmate, but the game goes on. Logic can set up all these walls to channel where we go, but in the middle of a discussion the other guy slips through the wall like a ghost. It doesn't do any good, I've come to understand, to complain: "Hey, that's against the rules." After all, whoever legislated that logical argument was to reign supreme in our lives?

I cherish what I learned from my father about the virtue of clarity and consistency. But I've also come to understand that my experience with him in the ways of rhetoric and persuasion did not teach me the whole picture about how we come to the understandings that move us in our lives. And so I've worked to expand my repertoire in the craft of persuasion, adding to the structure of my work music and complexity and indirection, even at the cost— sorry, Dad—of some of the crystalline clarity of an argument's progression.

But even words of the most powerful sort are but a rehearsal of the actual drama of life. "You had to be there" applies not just to getting some jokes, but to most of life's big lessons as well.

Starting in May 1963, I knew that my father was dying of cancer. This was something I thought about a great deal. My father and I discussed it extensively. He believed, as he liked to say, in grabbing the bull by the tail and looking the truth squarely in the face. I am—in that way, among others—my father's son. Denial is not our way. No cosmetics for the ugly truth.

On one of his visits to Cambridge, Massachusetts, to visit me, we went for a walk through the Commons. He was in good shape. It had been several months since his most recent bout had put him back into the hospital for another round of chemotherapy. I hadn't been there, but I understood from my mother that it was no picnic. (Or maybe I didn't "understand," but I had heard it.)

When I asked him how he was doing with the Hodgkin's, he gave me a little bit of medical reporting, and then added in a lower voice: "I'm afraid in a different way than I have been. A feeling of foreboding is getting more palpable. Can I tell you a dream?" We sat on a park bench.

"I had a dream last week that I was flying through a winter night sky above a frozen lake. But I wasn't in control of where I was flying—just propelled somehow. Soon I swooped down at the ice and struck it at a glancing angle, then bouncing off it back into the sky. Then again down at the ice, but at a slightly less acute angle, and bouncing up. And again. And finally, I was coming in and thinking this is too steep! Maybe the ice won't hold! And I hit the ice and broke through into the freezing water. I woke up absolutely terrified."

We discussed the dream, which he thought pretty transparent. The cycle of bouncing off the ice paralleled the cycling over the past three and a half years of bouts of pain and toxic treatments with intervals of more or less normal life albeit plagued with a higher level of pain than he usually let on. And as for the meaning of breaking through the ice? That wasn't too hard to find, either. "I'm afraid," Dad said, "that the dream says that this cycle doesn't just keep on going. That there's an end coming."

"It's perfectly natural, I think," I said, trying to be reassuring, though I couldn't say to which of us principally, "that you would be dreaming of death and your fear of time running out. But that doesn't mean that it's an accurate reflection of what's actually happening in the disease. I mean, people have nightmares that *don't* happen, too."

In the summer of 1967, my father's health began a sudden and steep descent. As I drove him to his radiation treatments, with him crouched in pain in the backseat of the car, we could both hear the clock ticking loudly for him. The treatments didn't produce the hoped-for respite, and soon he was in the hospital again. I was then in the process of moving from Cambridge to Chicago, but as soon as I could I came back to Minnesota to be with him, and with my mother, who was almost immobilized emotionally with dread. My brother flew in from California.

After I picked up Ed at the Minneapolis/St. Paul airport, we drove straight to the hospital for a briefing from my father's doctor. Actually, his usual doctor—Dr. Brown, a wonderful man—was out of town, and his place in supervising my father's treatment had been taken over by Dr. Green. Green was no Brown in terms of the human touch.

"You know, of course, your father's in desperate shape," Dr. Green told us. "The disease is moving quite rapidly. You'll probably notice that he isn't as alert as you remember him; I think the cancer is affecting his cognitive abilities. I wouldn't recommend you try to talk with him about what's going on; I doubt he'd understand it very well." When asked directly about his prognosis, and then about how long he had, Green answered: "We never know for sure, but I think we're talking about a matter of weeks at most."

When we left Green's office, Ed and I took a few minutes in the hospital corridor to try to pull ourselves together after Dr. Green's tactful discourse. I didn't know how much my tears were about the prospect, still theoretical, of losing Dad soon, and how much about the image of him at this moment no longer *compos mentis*. Dad without a sharp mind was hardly conceivable, would not even be Dad. Dad as pathetic, incapable of looking the facts squarely in the face, was a humiliating and painful image for me. (The next year, I recall, I had a dream mixing that scene with Dr. Green with the shots that killed JFK, and in the dream the line ran through my mind, "Dad-dead/Had-head.") Ed and I composed ourselves and went into Dad's room, ready to be cheerful.

After hugging Ed, whom he hadn't seen in months, Dad regarded me. "You look a little moist around the eyes and nose," he observed.

"Yeah, well, you know how my allergies are this time of year."

He knew we'd been to see Green. "How long have you been in the hospital? Half an hour? You know, they've got sophisticated air filters handling all the air in this place. So it isn't allergies." He paused, and looked at us both. "Boychicks, you shouldn't think that I don't know what's happening."

He was still Dad.

From the time I first learned about his cancer, I had more than four years to prepare for his death, and I used them as best I could. Even so, when he actually died in early October, slipping into a most final oblivion out of a raspy coma I found terrifying to hear and to see, I discovered I was in no way prepared for his death. It was one thing to imagine my life going on without my father; for him actually to be gone was an altogether different matter.

It was this experience, more than any other, that taught me how true it is that experience is the greatest teacher.

And a good thing it is, too, that it is experience more than any other force that shapes our core orientation to the world. What could be more trustworthy as an indication of what the world is really like than what we have actually lived of it? Words are wonderful, but by means of words we can be persuaded of notions that are not true. Thinking may be the crowning achievement of our species, but the saying "as quick as thought" suggests how loosely anchored can be the intellectual process in relation to our felt reality. Better to be rooted in the lessons engraved by real experience, working cumulatively over the course of our lives. The world must be that way, or at least part of it, or what happened wouldn't have happened. Long before our ancestors sprouted the crown of our neocortex, we were wired for learning knowledge of a still deeper kind out of the traumas and joys of our experience.

But experience also has its limits. How am I to comprehend truly the meaning of what has not yet happened? I hear that my father is dying, and the news makes a profound impression on me. But as profound as it is, it is superficial compared with actually witnessing his death and then proceeding to find him not there, again and again for the rest of my life. As an adolescent who could go for years at a time without missing school on account of illness, I knew that any person might be assailed by health problems; in the bloom of my vigor, however, my experience suggested to me that I was invincible. Rabbi Kushner knew that all kinds of terrible calamities happen to people, but it was only when a catastrophe befell his own family that he ever felt any need to reexamine his assumption of a God both omnipotent and just.[20]

"Real conviction in things human comes from experience and almost never through dialectics." So writes Bernard Berenson at the end of a rueful passage in which he remembers regretfully his previous incapacity to sympathize with his ill wife. "How in her last years my wife used to annoy me with her choking cough, her flusters, her tottering step. Why, because convinced [*sic*] they were controllable and if she would she could get the better of them. Now my own experience tells I did her wrong, that she could not help it. . . . Now that I too have to count my steps I recall with remorse the way I used to whip and drag her on."[21] Only with his own direct experience of illness did Berenson come to understand that the powers of a human being can fail, beyond his power to control.

If a loss is short-term, one might in some way disregard it, like some cartoon character who has walked past the edge of a cliff but does not fall because he does not yet recognize that there is nothing beneath him. Something like this seems to have been part of Joseph Heller's coping strategy in the face of his acute and devastating attack of Guillain-Barré syndrome. Doubtless Heller's approach is in part a function of his overall character structure. The author whose light way of confronting darkness I enjoyed so much when,

three decades ago, I read *Catch 22* was recognizable, in a bizarre
sort of way, when he says of the progressive and rapid loss of his
physical abilities: "The feeling was almost 'quaint.' " (Despite calling his account *No Laughing Matter,* Heller imbues the memoir
with a tone of playful levity.) I am certain that even with a short-
term health crisis, the author of *The Parable of the Tribes,* a work
conspicuously lacking in laughs, would never have described his
creeping paralysis as quaint; nor would that hypervigilant fellow
ever have shown Heller's uninquisitiveness when, sitting with his
doctor just before he began his siege in the hospital, he lost some of
his vital bodily functions: "I could not widen my jaws enough to
take a full-sized bite, could barely chew what I did manage to get
into my mouth, could not manipulate my tongue and throat into
swallowing what I did chew. Morty [his doctor] said nothing about
what he observed. He said nothing about Guillain-Barré. And I
didn't ask." But I wonder how long Heller could have persisted in
his characteristic style of defense had his disability proven truly
chronic and permanent. Consider his remarks about how his disease made him "cadaverously thin":

> I myself was oblivious to the change—until six months
> later, when I was out of the hospital and able to study
> myself in a mirror as I sat in my wheelchair in bathing
> trunks and a short-sleeved shirt. I was appalled by the
> extent to which I had withered. And by that time I had
> regained more than fifteen of the thirty or forty I'd
> lost.[22]

It is difficult to imagine him maintaining this stance of obliviousness if years went by without his ever regaining his health, his
capacities, his very flesh.

Time matters. Habits long-ingrained are not changed overnight.
The continual confrontation with my own chronic malady, I

could feel, was starting to change me at a deep level. Old habits die hard, but when the old way keeps on not working—when time after time it just leads to frustration—we eventually learn to let go.

For me, being capable had always been the keystone of the structure of my self-acceptance—being a can-do kind of guy. In my favorite picture of myself from my youth, taken in the hills of California in 1970, I looked like a young David ready to do battle with Goliath, which pretty well captures my stance toward the world in those years. Now my illness told me that, though Goliath is still out there, it would have to be others who would sling their stones at him. But that left me with a problem: if the exercise of my strength was how I justified my existence for the first forty-some years of my life, how was I to think myself okay when I was chronically weakened?

Since I have never liked failing, the repeated experiences of failing at the old game, I observed, were goading me to redefine the game. *Being good* at something seems less consequential, while just *being* seems like most of what there is.

I've spent much of my life wrestling with ambition, sometimes embracing it, driven by it. Sometimes wanting to be free of it, to be—like Chuang-tzu—disdainful of it. Now it seemed that my illness was teaching me, reluctant student that I was, a way to let go of it.

LET THAT BE A LESSON TO YOU

Illness can teach us of our vincibility. But how are we to learn of our mortality? This is one area in which experience seems quite inadequate as a teacher.

We all know that the world existed before us. But that time before our birth exists only hypothetically. We have no experience of our nonexistence, so how are we to imagine it? As for our death, that is always something—also quite hypothetical—presumed to await us out there in the future.

What about using the experience of others? To this, too, there are limits, and for precisely the same reason. Here is a Zen story:

> At the death of a parishioner, Master Dogo, accompanied by his disciple Zengen, visited the bereaved family. Without taking the time to express a word of sympathy, Zengen went up to the coffin, rapped on it, and asked Dogo, "Is he really dead?"
>
> "I won't say," said Dogo.
>
> "Well?" insisted Zengen.
>
> "I'm not saying, and that's final."
>
> On their way back to the temple, the furious Zengen turned on Dogo and threatened, "By God, if you don't answer my question, why, I'll beat you!"
>
> "All right, beat away."
>
> A man of his word, Zengen slapped his master a good one.
>
> Some time later, Dogo died, and Zengen, still anxious to have his question answered, went to the master Sekiso and, after relating what had happened, asked the same question of him.
>
> Sekiso, as if conspiring with the dead Dogo, would not answer.
>
> "By God," cried Zengen, "you too?"
>
> "I'm not saying, and that's final."
>
> At that very instant Zengen experienced an awakening.[23]

Indeed, the dead are not saying.

The concept "all men are mortal" gets daily support from the obituary column. None of the signers of the Declaration of Independence are among us now. Every single person in every photograph taken during the Civil War has, by now, perished. The grim implication is inescapable—but logic does not always grab us by the innards. Surely, it may be said, we all know death. Our world is permeated with it, and our collective imagination is haunted by it. But, once again, our knowledge can be just a cloak over our obliviousness.

In some ways, our "knowledge" of death may serve as the armor to protect our ignorance of its reality. In his book about the death of his parents, *The Time of Their Dying,* Stephen Rosenfeld of the *Washington Post* reports his discovery that "it was possible to live in a century in which death has been dealt out by men on a scale never before contemplated, and to work in a business, newspapering, in which death is a routine part of the job (I broke in, the typical cub, on obits), and yet to have seen death only at a distance denying a true, felt knowledge of it."[24] As for the murderous mayhem that pervades our mass media, Johann Hofmeier directly rebuts the idea that the representations of death to which we are exposed would serve to encourage a deeper emotional experience of the reality of death among people in modern society. The film reports we so often see, he asserts, "seem to deaden rather than awaken feeling for [the] underlying content." And the standard patterns of films—"in which the figure with whom the audience can identify is successful, confident and immune from death"— "strengthen a person's existing illusion of his own immortality and thereby counteract any experience of death."[25] Similarly, Kavanaugh writes in *Facing Death* that "television feeds our fantasy of forever being a spectator." What is the effect on us of seeing so many images we know to be mere fantasy? From his experience at witnessing the parade of deaths in the media, Kavanaugh concludes, "Even a bloody nose or a fainting spell by a fellow viewer would have aroused more emotion in me than a hundred deaths on the tube."[26]

Our species' gift for making symbols—developing languages, creating artworks, performing mathematical manipulations—both strengthens and weakens our hold on reality. It gives us powers to reshape the world around us, but it can also make our grasp of what is real more tenuous. Just as we can know and not know something, so can the images before our eyes seem real and not real at the same time. When our car goes out of control, and we seem to be gliding toward disaster, we are likely to feel we are somehow suddenly enacting some scene in a movie. While at one level our imaginative fantasies can serve as rehearsals for real experience, at another level they create an emotional space for playing with experiences whose reality we can deny. Stewart Alsop recounts his experience in meeting with an old friend and a broker to confer "solemnly" about the changed financial prospects for his family

> given the statistical probability that I would be dead in a year or a bit more.
> We were calm and businesslike as we counted up my assets . . . and so on. It gave me an odd sense of unreality—it was hard to grasp that it was, after all, *my* death we were discussing so rationally, and I had a feeling that we were three characters in a rather bad play.[27]

We watch death all the time, but it is almost as though it were a vaccination against having to deal with a "live" version of the affliction.

Do we know that we will die? There are some who have argued that we do not—that, in fact, we *cannot*—really know. In a much-cited passage, Freud argued that

> it is indeed impossible to imagine our own death: and whenever we attempt to do so we can perceive that we are in fact still present as spectators. Hence the psychoan-

alytic school could venture on the assertion that at bottom no one believes in his own death, or, to put the same thing in another way, that in his unconscious, every one of us is convinced of his own immortality.[28]

Similarly, the Roman philosopher Lucretius argued that one who indulges in self-pity at the thought of his body's destiny after death "unconsciously . . . is making some vestige of himself survive." Lucretius does not, like Freud, argue that *every* person unconsciously believes in his immortality. His argument about the unconscious assumption of the persistence of our awareness is in service of his overriding point that death is nothing to fear; it is specifically to the fearful person that he attributes the failure "to see that, in real death, he will have no second self that will be still alive and capable of lamenting to itself over its own death, or of grieving, as he stands, in imagination, over his prostrate self, that he is being mangled by beasts of prey or being cremated."[29]

This image of a grisly fate awaiting one's corpse reminds me of one of the more powerful experiences I have had in the process of working on this book. I read Brigham Young's request concerning the specifications for his coffin. What he wanted, he said, was a coffin that was

> from two to three inches wider than is commonly made for a person of my breadth and size, and deep enough to place me on a little comfortable cotton bed, with a good suitable pillow for size and quality; the coffin to have the appearance that if I wanted to turn a little to the right or left I should have plenty of room to do so.

As I first reflected on this passage, I felt a sense of condescending amusement at Brigham Young's concerns: what the hell difference does it make? Doesn't he know that he won't be doing any turning around? Then, as the image settled a little deeper into my mind, I was suddenly filled with panic. Picturing myself in a coffin, regardless of its dimensions, gave me the same fright I recall feeling as a boy when, crawling through an underground tunnel dug by a friend of mine, I pictured the ground collapsing upon me. Imagine being trapped underground for eternity! The thought left me shaken.

Suddenly, the original question about our knowledge of our mortality appears to have been stood upon its head. Instead of the original concern—is it not embarrassing to treat as important the quite obvious proposition that "all men (and women) are mortal"?—it seems we have to confront the opposite possibility: is it not futile to concern ourselves with the unimaginable notion that each of us will die?

I think it is not futile, for just as there are different levels of knowledge, so also are there different degrees of unimaginability. We are not all of us all the time equally out of touch with the reality of our mortality. Leaving for later in this work the question of what is the value of experiencing—or even cultivating—an awareness of death, let us look at some of the ways that we can come to be less ignorant of the reality of our being mortal creatures.

CLOSER TO HOME

The deaths of others may not always be real when we see them on the tube, but some deaths do strike us with a force great enough to change us. While Rosenfeld found that he had been able to work as a newspaperman for years without developing "a true, felt knowledge" of death, it was through undergoing the demise of his parents that he realized the superficiality of his previous knowledge. Similarly Ben Hecht tells the event that precipitated his conscious-

ness from one of presumed indestructibility to one where he knows
he is mortal. "I can recall the hour in which I lost my immortality,
in which I tried on my shroud for the first time and saw how it
became me. . . . The knowledge of my dying came to me when
my mother died."[30] Though there is a boundary of sorts between
self and other, the boundary is quite permeable. Some people—by
virtue of the bonds of love and identification—we experience as
standing within the bounds of the self, and so their deaths are felt as
a death of part of ourselves. When death hits close to home, we
become that much more persuaded that what remains of us also lies
in death's domain.

While it is true that, until we die, we can have no complete
experience of death, some experiences can bring the knowledge
home. In his discussion of how little we know of death as something appertaining to our own lives, Josef Mayer Scheu nonetheless
notes the possibility of transformative experiences in our relation
with death. "If I cross a main road carelessly and a lorry hurtles by
just in front of me, I experience death for a moment as one aware
of it. If I allow myself to become fully conscious of this experience,
. . . after moments like that life looks quite different."[31]

And then there is that teacher with which I began—illness.
Stewart Alsop learned from his leukemia. He had occasion before
his illness to know about mortality, but, he says, "If you are young
and in good spirits and full of health, the thought of dying is not
only utterly abhorrent but inherently incredible." Even being terminally ill can seem unreal if it stays at the level of "news," and
never enters the realm of felt experience. Kenneth Shapiro, for
example, still found it incredible that he was dying, even after being
told by all the medical authorities that his cancer gave him but a
short time to live, because his moment-to-moment experience was
still one of good health and spirits. "Here I am, supposedly dying
and I don't feel bad. . . . That being the case, I have always found

it very hard to accept the fact that I am supposed to be dying, and my gut reaction was, no I am not dying."[32] For him, the news remains not impotent—even being missed by a lorry can have an impact—but still somewhat hypothetical. Stewart Alsop's previous confrontation with death had been as a soldier in World War II, where he felt strong and healthy, but was living in a situation in which, as it were, lorries were continuously rushing at him. "[T]he fear of death in battle is quite different from the fear of death on a hospital bed," writes Alsop from his hospital bed. "Sickness and age do not make death at all incredible."

And so, too, has my experience of illness diminished my incredulity in the face of this obvious, unwelcome, and unimaginable truth.

OFF AND ON

Big things are hard to carry without intermittent rests. Just as one who walks with a heavy suitcase is apt to set it down at intervals to regather strength, so will a person needing to bear some momentous news likely need interruptions in the knowing and the acknowledging of the heavy tidings.

To some extent, this intermittency of knowing probably applies to good news as well as bad. If I were to win the ten million dollars that my mail from Ed McMahon sometimes tantalizingly suggests I already have won, that would be good news, relieving me as it would of numerous worries and uncertainties. Yet I expect that— just as John D. Rockefeller persisted throughout his life as a multimillionaire in stashing potatoes around his house as provision against the still-felt threat of starvation—I would *know* I was rich only some of the time, while continuing at other times to feel that prudence required me to buy my winter coats at yard sales. Even if good news can be difficult to integrate into one's moment-to-moment perspective, however, the problem is even greater when the news is painful and catastrophic, as with the recognition that one has irretrievably lost a loved one, or the knowledge that eventually, if not sooner, one will lose everything through one's own death.

The night my father died, there were moments when the impact of recognizing what had happened was almost more than I could bear. That impact was certainly more than I was willing to bear continually. When we got home at around four in the morning, my brother and I stayed up to play the game of Twixt, an engrossing contest of strategy our father had introduced to us the previous year. For a few seconds at a time, focusing our minds on the configurations on the board was a perfect escape from the pain of confronting the knowledge that night had thrust upon us.

C. S. Lewis, in his moving journal about his grief over the death of his wife, describes his own intermittent fleeing from the full recognition of the magnitude of his loss. Where my brother and I distracted ourselves with intellectualizing, Lewis sought solace by rationalizing. "There are moments," Lewis wrote,

> most unexpectedly, when something inside me tries to assure me that I don't really mind so much, after all. Love is not the whole of a man's life. I was happy before I ever met H. I've plenty of what are called "resources". People get over these things. Come, I shan't do so badly. One is ashamed to listen to this voice but it seems for a little to be making out a good case. Then comes a sudden jab of red-hot memory and all this "commonsense" vanishes like an ant in the mouth of a furnace.[33]

There is nothing pathological about this alternation of escape with recognition. In her book *The Courage to Grieve,* Judy Tatelbaum writes that this movement "in and out of pain" is natural, and she suggests that those coping with such loss should allow themselves this intermittency. "The natural process of grieving," she says, "involves experiencing times of intense feeling and then following them with periods of quiet."[34]

As with the loss of a loved one, so also with accepting one's own death.

In her famous and pioneering work on the dying process, Elisabeth Kübler-Ross identified *denial* as the first stage that people go through when they are brought face-to-face with their impending death. "It can't be true. This isn't happening to me." In time, Kubler-Ross said, people can work through their denial, as well as other intermediate stages, and gain *acceptance*.

Others since then have maintained that people do not so much pass through these stages in a sequential order as weave their way in and out of them. A "hive effect," Shneidman calls it, with "constant coming and going."[35] A young man dying of cancer says that all the stages are part of each day. This young man, whose voice is heard in Kleinman's *Illness Narratives,* tells us of his offs and ons: "Today I can't accept it [my death]. Yesterday I did partly. Saturday, I was there: kind of in a trance, waiting, ready to die. But not now."[36] Sometimes the dying person acknowledges the inevitable, sometimes seeks refuge in "disbelief and hope."[37] Again, it is only natural. "It is only human," says Shneidman, "for even the most extraordinary human beings occasionally to blot out or take a vacation from their knowledge of their imminent end."[38]

My own end does not seem particularly imminent. I am not dying in any sense save that in which it is true for all of us. But, as I've said, spending such an extended period of time with my own personal kryptonite within me has sufficiently disabused me of the belief that I am Superman that I've come to accept in my guts that I am mortal. That is, now and then I face the knowledge that I will die. The rest of the time, I skate along on our customary thin ice as if it were terra firma. As if now were forever, as if time would not inevitably bring on the season of my nonbeing.

Even while trying as best I could to look the facts of my mortality squarely in the face, I discovered myself playing other games. While developing this project—which is, in large measure, an exercise in putting myself in perspective—I caught myself making a ludicrous ploy to preserve my comforting illusions. Lurking in the corner, I spied the tacit hope that—like the ancients at their altars—I might spare myself the fate the gods have in mind for me by making the proper sacrifice. What was ludicrous was my subconscious proposition to the gods: the idea is that by sacrificing my comforting and tacit illusions about my immortality, by laying my firstborn pride out on the altar, I might manage to get *my life* spared.

THIS IS IT!

" ' " ' "We all die," said that woman whose wisdom Solomon praises in the Book of Kings.' " [The professor, looking up from his reading of an earlier thinker] let his big hand fall on the desk, paused for effect, and remarked, "She was quite an original thinker, that woman." ' "[39]

This is from a complex passage in Ariès's *The Hour of Our Death*. Quotes within quotes within quotes, a cascade through French history representing a sequence of attitudes. The earliest French speaker, quoting the woman said to be praised by Solomon, is Bousset, to whom the idea that "we all die" was important and meaningful. Then comes the professor, Bellesoort, whose mocking of Bousset is recalled approvingly by his student, Pierre-Henri Simon, who is telling the story. To the professor and his student, the pronouncement deemed wise by Bousset seems "pompous and trite." The final voice, overseeing this evolution of attitudes from speaker to speaker, each reflecting "the context of his age," is

Ariès. Ariès's posture is ostensibly the dispassionate one of the scientific student of history. But the nuances of his language—characterizing Bousset as having "understood," and saying that Bellesoort's humorous portrayal came "despite [his] education and goodwill"—suggests that Ariès finds more wisdom than pomposity in the statement "We all die."

A case can be made for either position. The statement is certainly *not* original. But is it trite? My point is: we cannot know from the words alone. Words are but signs—sometimes they point to profoundly felt meanings and understandings, sometimes they are mere words. The difference between a platitude and a profundity lies in the essential and sacred realm of experience. Like many sacred realms, this one is invisible: it is not the visible letter but the invisible spirit that distinguishes the trite from the revelatory.

Even the obvious can strike with the force of revelation, being no less a revelation for being obvious.

Back in the days of the psychedelic subculture, a story circulated about a young man who had an intense trip one night in Hawaii. At one point, it was said, he felt he had discovered the essential truth of life. He rushed to write it down, lest he might lose forever, once the psychedelic state had worn off, the vital truth that had been vouchsafed him. The next day, he went with great expectation to read his sacred text from the night before. On the paper were written the words "This is It!"

As I recall, the story was told to point out the illusory nature of the sense of revelation and profundity that one could experience in that altered state of consciousness: the guy thought he had some big truth, the story was deemed to show, but he really had nothing.

But I see it otherwise. As a sacred text, I admit, "This is It!" is not of much use. I suspect, however, that the young man, however inarticulate at that crucial moment, was right about his realization of that moment: "This"—whatever it was—probably is at least an important piece of "It!"

CHAPTER 4

Tethered to a Dying Animal

Putting Ourselves in Perspective

NOT ME

A Yiddish saying expresses the craziness I have discerned in myself. "Dear God, you do wonderful things for complete strangers. So why not me?"

The assumption that I must occupy a special place in God's universe, as I do in my own, seriously undercut when my plans for my life were derailed by illness. That sort of thing might happen to complete strangers, but not to me. According to this implicit view of the cosmos, with a pre-Copernican narcissistic self at the center, my vital powers should go on flowering. If that's what my life is about, I seem to feel in my inner heart, that should be a law of the natural order.

Had I been killed instantly in a car crash, my narcissistic assumptions would have been violated, but I never would have had occasion to revise my cosmology. The experience of outliving myself compelled me to reexamine my place in the great scheme of things.

Looking into the human encounter with our finitude, I discover that, in thinking myself special, I am no different from other people. "In a hundred years, we shall all be dust—but not I," says Scheu, speaking in the voice of Everyman.[1] "All men think all men mortal but themselves," wrote the seventeenth-century English poet Edward Young.[2] Young would not have been surprised at the difficulty experienced by Ivan Ilyich, Tolstoy's famous dying character, in discovering that the prototypical syllogism applies to him. The inescapable trap—"All men are mortal"—which was shown to me as snaring Socrates, Ilyich evidently learned with death capturing Caius.

> That Caius—man in the abstract—was mortal, was perfectly correct, but he was not Caius, not an abstract man, but a creature quite separate from all others. . . . "Caius really was mortal, and it was right for him to die; but for me, little Vanya, Ivan Ilych, with all my thoughts and emotions, it's altogether a different matter."[3]

When we are struck by the obvious, part of the blow is evidently a narcissistic injury. Here is one additional obstacle to our knowing what is logically manifest and inescapable. Not only is it hard to give reality to what we have never experienced. Not only do we have motive to deny the prospect of loss that would, in any event, be painful. But we have, most of us, a need to be more important in the great scheme of things than we actually are. I am not "man in the abstract," I am me, with my special and irreplaceable store of treasures. Little Vanya, being special, should be exempt from the iron law of the human condition.

Dear God, I understand you have to inflict tragedies on complete strangers, but certainly not me. "This can't be happening to me," writes Thomas Bell of his coming to grips with his malignant tumor. *"Me* with only a few months to live? Nonsense." He goes on:

> Perhaps the difficulty is my half-conscious presumption that such things happen, should happen, only to other people. . . . People who are strangers, who really don't mind, who . . . are born solely to fill such quotas. Whereas I am me. Not a stranger. Not other people. Me![4]

Confronting my illness gradually moved from that question one often hears from the afflicted, "Why me?," to the question my aunt Chava raised. My father's sister, she has gone through life with much the same attitude about grabbing the bull by the tail as her brother. After she was diagnosed with cancer, she considered her situation and asked: "Why not me?"

EMBODIMENT

"If the body, monks, were the self," reads one of the sutras of the Buddhist literature, "the body would not be subject to disease."[5] I make no pretense to be an expert in Buddhism, nor to be privy to whatever ultimate truth there may be about the human self. But despite my respect for Buddhist wisdom and my acknowledgment of my own ignorance, I must say that I find the logic of this sutra far from persuasive. There is a premise here, left unstated as if it were self-evident: that there is a part of a person that must be enduring and immutable. That's a comforting thought, but is there any reason to believe it?

However lacking in foundation the premise may be, it is consistent with what I called my pre-Copernican narcissistic view of the cosmos. In this view, it was an insult that when something went amiss in my guts, my spirit also lost its zest. Just because of a problem with my *body*, the life of my *mind* became crippled. Evidently I still thought my real self was above all that.

Yeats has a phrase: "tethered to a dying animal." My illness made the phrase meaningful to me. My mind was in no apparent sense free of my body. If the animal body that I am felt poisoned, my mind felt toxic, too. I had formerly thought like a healthy animal. Now I was thinking like an ill one. The intimate connection between mind and body is not altogether a new discovery for me. What is somewhat new is discerning the sorrowful dimension of the one being tethered to the other.

When I was a youth, quite interested in depth psychology, I was resistant to perspectives that stressed the role of the material realm in governing our psychological and spiritual aspects. The issue seemed to me part of the larger struggle in our civilization between a view of our nature that honors our humanity and one that attempts to reduce us to the status merely of sophisticated machines. That was how I saw, for example, the controversy between those stressing the value of psychotherapy in helping people deal with problems in their emotional lives and those who emphasize treatment with drugs. I saw the pharmacological approach as an expression of that force in our culture that, with its reductionistic vision, reduces the human being to a paltry mechanism.

In some respects, my values have not changed. I still regard the human mind and spirit as wondrous and deserving of our deep attention. I still believe that what we think and feel shapes our experience and our very world in profound ways. And I still believe that our humanity is threatened by systems of understanding that look at us as if through the wrong end of a powerful telescope.

But I no longer believe that our experience is separable from our chemistry. Where I formerly imagined myself as living *in* my body, I now would say I *am* my body.

"All day, all night," writes Virginia Woolf in her essay "On Being Ill," "the body intervenes . . . The creature within can only gaze through the pane, smudged or rosy."[6]

How many me's are there? Montaigne seems to have at least three. He complains that his mind "has picked up such a close friendship with my body that, when the body calls, it deserts me at every turn." Who is the "me" who is deserted? Nothing, I would say, but his desire to be in a state of fitness better than he finds himself. That is a desire I know well. "Somehow," Montaigne continues, "if [my mind's] comrade comes down with a fit of colic, down it comes too."[7] We would wish, like the Buddhist of the sutra, to have as one's real address some impregnable fortress, and have the body a mere recreational escape, like a beach house one might sell off when times get rough. But it seems to me we have but one home, with no change of address possible. I am one me, pitched by the sea, beaten upon by wind and waves, in varying states of disrepair.

REVOLTING ANIMAL

To discover that one's consciousness is a function of the body can be an injury to one's narcissism not just because the body goes the way of all flesh. There is also a problem with how we feel about animals of flesh and blood.

Saint Paul sided with his willing spirit against the flesh, whose inclinations he regarded as weakness. Between the angels and the beasts, the Renaissance saw us, with the bestial aspect of our natures of course being the lower and regrettable part. Ernest Becker characterizes us as "gods with anuses." An unbridgeable split, a polarization—just the kind of structure one would expect in an image essentially narcissistic in nature. For the narcissist feels himself simultaneously superior and inferior, deified and humiliated.

In my two principal works on the evolution of civilization, I explore at some length the origins of the war against our inborn nature as human creatures and the dynamics of the narcissistic project by which we seek to repair the damage to our self-respect inflicted by civilized cultures imbued with some profoundly antihuman values. Here, suffice it to say that living in civilized society gives us a pressing reason to wish to be able to transcend what we have received from nature: such transcendence can seem the best strategy for making peace with the cultural forces that bear down upon us.

In the vortex of an ongoing war between civilization, with its demands, and nature, with its incredibly complex living structures, the very processes that make possible the blessings of life can come to be regarded as loathsome and repulsive. That "we are born between urine and faeces," Freud said, is something to which we take exception.[8]

> *There is naught but filthiness,*
> *Mucus, spittle, rottenness,*
> *Stinking rotten excrement.*
> *Consider the products of nature . . .*
> *You will see that each man brings*
> *Stinking matter, loathsome things*
> *From his body constantly.*[9]

So wrote the poet Nesson. And countless other images of the body as stinking stuff, "a bag of dung," could be adduced from the heritage of our Western spiritual traditions. While in our culture, sexuality and excretion are the special targets of shame, in other cultures it can be other aspects of our animality. In the Balinese society described by Clifford Geertz, for example, it is eating. We are not content to be healthy animals, eating and eliminating and reproducing. Against our animal nature, which we are taught to regard as revolting, we revolt.

If a healthy animal is bringing forth loathsome things constantly, how much worse is a diseased one? Illness is another and most unwelcome reminder of our animal nature. Illness reduces a person; it can magnify the essentials of living into the main event: Can you hold your food down? Are you able to eat enough? Are your trips to the toilet successful? Can you get enough breath? These are animal issues. And to the extent one has incorporated a cultural attitude of repulsion toward our animal natures, to that extent will the injury of illness be compounded by the insult of having one's nose rubbed into the falseness of one's narcissistic self-image.

SAY IT AIN'T SO, CAELIA

> *Nor wonder how I lost my Wits;*
> *Oh! Caelia, Caelia, Caelia shits!*[10]

In this couplet by the great Irish author Jonathan Swift, we see another side of the narcissistic project to transcend one's condition. Instead of the "Not me" that would insist on being, oneself, an exception to the rules governing human life, there is a "Not you" directed toward the one who embodies one's idealized aspirations. One may presume that the speaker who is horror-struck at Caelia's bodily practices is daily reminded that he does the same.

The words of Swift, of course, cannot be assumed to give voice to the feelings of Everyman: by any standard, Jonathan Swift was a strange man, with his own rather intense discomforts with corporeality. Yet neither are the feelings he reports wholly idiosyncratic. When Norman O. Brown draws on that couplet of Swift, and on others of his writings about the body (in a chapter Brown entitles

"The Excremental Vision"), he ventures that Swift, for all his individual peculiarities, is making manifest a "universal neurosis."

I can understand Swift's incredulity about Caelia. To me, also, it has seemed that the loveliness of a beautiful woman should confer some immunity from the pitfalls of our animal bodies. When Grace Kelly died in a car accident caused, reportedly, by her suffering a stroke while driving, I found myself surprised—as well as surprised by my surprise—that such a beauty could be extinguished by the bursting of a blood vessel in her brain. And, more recently, when Audrey Hepburn died of cancer of the colon, there was a part of me that found it difficult to believe that so lovely a creature as appeared in *Roman Holiday* could have a colon at all, much less one with malignant tumors growing in it.

But my resonance with Swift's lament about Caelia doesn't prove Brown's point about his universality. I'm no Everyman, either; rather I'm the product of a particular upbringing, one that might suggest that my observation of myself should not permit me to take the leap and speak of "our" failure to integrate the reality of our animal bodies with our idealized image of the human being.

My ancestral culture labored to channel much of the energy of the body into the precincts of the mind. My father, in his focus on mental energy, was certainly an embodiment (if that's the word) of that cultural tendency: in his head, not well grounded in his body.

My mother is a more down-to-earth person. Of her contributions to forming my worldview, among the most cherished is the marvelous way she has infused her ideals for human life with the most basic human values. The people she would hold up to us as most admirable were those who, whatever their station or their level of sophistication, possessed a core of virtue and character. Her stories were of wise peasant women and of the peddler of pretzels on the street in Philadelphia who always had time for a kind word and a playful joke for a poor girl like her. When she retired from her work as a high school teacher, the janitors and secretaries created an event, unusual for such retirements, to bid a special goodbye to her, for she was a teacher who treated the lower-level staff with the same respect as the professional. She was down-to-earth in that way—but, when it came to the body, she brought into our family some culture of prudish discomfort. More than just privacy, a curtain of shame seemed to surround some aspects of our bodily existence. Between excessive intellectuality and prudery, therefore, I could easily believe that my own difficulties with integrating the body into the ideal were idiosyncratic rather than necessarily representative.

But "representativeness" is rather more complex than simple similarity. And it seems to be a general human tendency—if not always in the exactly identical way—to construct ideals that transcend the animal realities of our human condition.

More than human. It is a phrase whose frequent repetition bespeaks its importance in our imaginative lives. Yet to what or whom does it refer? Has anyone actually encountered such a being, or is it simply a figment of our aspiration? If something more than human did not exist, we would have to invent it.

Among the Greeks, all that differentiated the gods from the humans was the extent of their powers and their immunity from death. The image of God in the monotheistic religions of Judaism and Christianity and Islam represents a more comprehensive departure from the human circumstance. This God has no need even for ambrosia, nor does He sneak around behind the back of a jealous wife to consummate His lust for various mortals.

Whether it be the God of heaven or a goddess, like the previously imagined Caelia who is "above" the sordid bodily functions of mere mortals, the idealized image represents the powers and traits in which one wishes somehow to participate. Thus the prophet imitates Jehovah's righteous wrath; the ascetic strives to imitate Christ's perfection; the lover seeks to complete himself with the human goddess who will raise him above his tawdry everyday life.

"Say it ain't so, Joe," said the boy in his famous encounter with his hero, Shoeless Joe Jackson, disgraced by the Black Sox scandal in professional baseball earlier in this century. The boy's anguish reflected genuine injury, for a model of what kind of man he might become had been damaged, and with it perhaps the chances of his ever attaining those betrayed ideals.

I once studied tragedy. Now I do the grocery shopping for my family, and in the checkout lines I read the headlines on the various tabloids. In literary terms, of course, the two are worlds apart. In psychological terms, however, I sense similar forces at play. Both deal with the exalted, and both bring them low. The child may need his heroes perfect—the unvanquished Heracles, the unsullied Shoeless Joe—but the adult has a more ambivalent relation with perfection. The adult is more compelled to temper aspiration with the reality of limitation. Tragedy and tabloid, one might venture, are both ways for common people to come to terms with their common humanity.

More than human—a king like Oedipus or Caesar, a princess like Di—yet also subject to the inescapable tribulations of the human condition. Tragedy and tabloid both build idols, and both expose the feet of clay. Tragedy—in Athens and Elizabethan England alike—deals not with the common person but with the most elevated, with royalty and with mythic heroes. Into their mouths it puts the most exalted speech, words of nobility and beauty, the finest the greatest poets can craft. And then it shows them in failure, defeat, and death; it shows them flawed and humbled, vulnerable to all the misfortunes to which flesh is heir.

Likewise the tabloids. They draw upon our pantheon of the

more than human. We see the richest (Donald Trump), the most glamorous (Marilyn Monroe still appears now and then in the tabloids' front page headlines), the most talented. The tabloids worship and humble them, at once declaring them worth our collective attention and revealing how all their money and glory cannot protect them against heartbreak. We read of Lady Di's bulimia, of Liz's latest diet, of one star or another having been molested as a child, or discovering that her husband is cheating on her.

At their core, both tragedy and tabloid reflect ambivalence. Lady Di is both made into a goddess and shown to be wretched. The hero is both more than we, and brought lower than we. At turns worshiped and pitied.

Part of this ambivalence might be understood in political terms. Something like the fattening of the sacrificial animal is occurring. In *Microcosm*, Philip Slater writes about how groups build up the king or leader in order later to feed upon his power. The bigger he is, the more to feed upon. Thus the tabloids and the tragedians both magnify and devour their heroes, cutting them into a thousand sacramental chunks for the throng to partake of. Both genres are expressions of the democratic spirit, part of the dissemination of sovereignty from the central crown to the empowered masses. It is not coincidence that the places where tragedy flowered—fifth-century Athens and Elizabethan England—were the places in the ancient and modern world where the idea of democracy gained its impetus. Nor is it just chance, I would suggest, that it is in our contemporary democracies that tabloids adorn the newsstands and checkout counters. A leveling process is at work, in which royalty is brought lower and the common man gains in power.

At a deeper level, however, more pertinent to our present concern, the ambivalence reflects the struggle between both knowing and not knowing the reality of our human condition. As with the mathematician's proof that builds upon the "limiting case," these forms of combined hero worship and iconoclasm provide proof that the human condition is indeed inescapable. If it is true even of Caelia, then it must be true of everyone. If even the stars are brought down to earth, then there must be no way out of our earthbound state. If the greatest must suffer, surely we must suffer, too.

More than human. We look at the limiting cases and realize there is no such thing. This realization helps us come to terms with our lives and face them more realistically. When Magic Johnson announces that he has HIV, those who idolize him discover that he is not a god. But the discovery goes beyond that. If even Magic Johnson can get HIV, many of the youths whose hero he was concluded, then I must be vulnerable, too. And I'd better adjust my ways accordingly.

In the literature on the saints, there are accounts of the flesh of the saints not decomposing in the usual way. One of the criteria for beatification, writes Ariès, was the "preservation of the body and the sweetness of its odor. The body of the saint is not subject to the universal corruption or its physical horrors."[11] I've not been in the presence of any of these incorruptible bodies, but I have my doubts. It seems as probable as that Caelia would differ in her food-processing methods from the usual mammalian technique. A more mature view of the fate of the flesh of a saint, it seems to me, is that found in Dostoyevsky's *The Brothers Karamazov*. In that novel, when the beloved and saintly Father Sossima dies, the character Alyosha is as disturbed as the disillusioned lover of Caelia when the corpse begins to emit a terrible stench. But in both cases, the losing of one's "wits" might well be a step toward gaining greater wisdom.

The psychoanalyst Otto Rank discussed how the genius "repeats the narcissistic inflation of the child," entertaining the fantasy that, by doing work "qualifying for immortality," he can exercise "control of life and death, of destiny, in the 'body' of his work."[12] If one's work is only great enough, the fantasy goes, one will gain entry into a special genus of beings: the immortals.

"We do not know of any immortals who existed before the absurdly brief time-span of oral and written history," writes Ira Wallach. He is skeptical of how long today's "immortals" will be immortal. But in any event, has anything important changed in terms of what it means to live a human life, just because one's work might now be preserved after one's death? Wallach says, "The only time one can enjoy one's immortality is when one is alive."[13]

We are not saved even by works, I remind myself as I listen to a Mozart aria of unearthly beauty. Mozart wrote music that was out of this world, I think, and then I remember that scene at the end of *Amadeus* when his body is unceremoniously dumped into a pit in the earth, excavated for the burial of paupers, and sprinkled with lye.

Even the immortals are mortal.

Ups and Downs: Thoughts on the Life Cycle

"The incredible shrinking man," I thought while, at 135 pounds, I stacked up the boxes for our move to the mountains. "No wonder I've been shying away from collisions on the basketball court: I'm not bringing much mass to the occasion (except maybe the kind of mass that begins with a *Kyrie Eleison*)." I recalled that I'd weighed 135 before, but not since I was in the seventh grade. It had felt rather different then. One hundred thirty-five pounds felt like a lot when I was first donning my muscle of manhood. Now I discovered that I was to have my doff days as well as my don days.

The wheel turns, and the way up feels quite different from the way down. Time is not always a friend. Eventually, it leaves us in the dust. It comes as a shock to really get it that we are tied to a cycle of time with downs as well as ups.

I reminded myself that this is hardly my first experience of how time brings changes. Growing up is filled with changes as life unfolds its blueprint for the developing creature. Every year bigger, more mature. But experiencing all that growth does not give intimation of the full picture. The first half is a coming into one's own, life handing out more and more equipment—size, strength, status. But eventually "the Lord giveth" turns into "the Lord taketh away," and having come into one's own does not really prepare one for going into one's disown.

My dispossession at that time—twenty pounds stripped from my frame—was of course somewhat ahead of schedule. But however premature was this indication that life has a postmature stage, I was starting to get the point.

I wonder if our outlook would be much different if life ran in reverse, if we began on our deathbed instead of a delivery table, if we started out old and decrepit and eventually became immature and incompetent, if instead of ending up food for worms we at last broke up into a sperm and an ovum. In some ways it would be a different kind of life cycle, but the pattern would still entail a waxing and then a waning.

Waxing is a heady feeling. On the way up, it seems as though one could go on forever. No young man thinks he will ever die, Hazlitt wrote.[14] The tendency of adolescents to see themselves as immortal is widely noted. Ben Hecht says that the young man he used to be "inhabited a world that was unthinkable without him. . . . He felt a childish immortality within the day he occupied."[15] Such an illusion can, of course, be dangerous. "Many young gays carry a conviction of indestructibility along with the belief, held at their peril, that AIDS is no threat to them."[16] But perhaps a degree of recklessness in the newly mature has been adaptive for the human primate group as a whole. Civilized societies make use of these adolescent illusions to man their armies—those who feel themselves indestructible willingly march off into battle. But perhaps in primitive societies as well the survival of the community was buttressed by the willingness of a corps of bold and dispensable members willing to take risks greater than rational calculation on purely individual terms would dictate.

Whatever the macrocosmic reason for this tendency in youth, the question still arises as to how it works psychologically. One possible interpretation is that denial is at work. Stillian and Wass, for example, say about the finding that 75 percent of adolescents "shut the idea of death out of their minds": "Adolescents may clothe themselves in an illusion of invulnerability in order to deny anxiety brought about by their mature understanding of death."[17] But that leaves the question why older people, also presumably with a mature understanding of death, do not clothe themselves so thoroughly in the same illusion. The reason, I suggest, may be that adolescents, having experienced only the waxing part of the life cycle, have less experiential basis for grasping the essential temporariness of human life.

It is only as one passes over the hill that the way down becomes visible. If there is a tendency for people to hit a bump on the road at midlife, perhaps this is why. An early proponent of the idea of the midlife crisis, Elliot Jacques, suggested that underlying this crisis is "the recognition of one's mortality and finitude."[18] Decline comes as a sort of revelation. What strikes terror in a person's heart, says James Dickey, is a photograph of oneself from the past: "You look at it and you know you are going to die."[19] A man in his forties reported to Judith Viorst, working on her book *Necessary Losses,* how a case of tennis elbow precipitated a crisis of anxiety. He became so worried, he says, "that I actually took the time to review my life insurance, though I know that tennis elbow is rarely fatal."[20]

One loses one's immortality before one loses one's life. Perhaps this is why the fear of death is reported to be greater at life's midpoint than at the end.[21]

Ed and I were discussing midlife as we worked together chopping wood. He was visiting me at my place in the mountains early in April, and he was enjoying the early-spring squall of snow that blew in. A Californian for the past thirty years, he didn't see snow very often. Ed was suggesting that my malady might be some kind of somatic midlife crisis.

"Midlife may be a time when life forces you to make some changes," said Ed, a clinical psychologist with a mystical bent. "Whatever wasn't right in one's approach to the first half has gotta change; it just doesn't work. Sometime around in your forties, the body says, 'You need to make a midcourse correction.' Maybe you make it, maybe you don't. Maybe it's the correct correction, maybe it's not."

"For the men in our family," I observed, "the forties certainly proved a tough decade." In addition to my problems, Ed had gone through a lot with his psoriatic arthritis, an autoimmune disorder that had taken a big toll on his comfort. And Dad, of course, never made it out of his forties. Ed shares my taste for gallows humor. So, I joked with him about seeing Dad's Hodgkin's in terms of Ed's notion of a midlife midcourse correction, reminding him of a line that used to crack me up in high school: "Death is nature's way of telling us it is time to slow down."

We stacked the wood and put away our axes, and took off toward the hot tub to soothe our not-so-young-anymore joints. "I'd like to think you're right about that midcourse correction business and my health problems; it implies that I'm not stuck, just in transition. Maybe it's like the convulsive shaking the pilots felt when they hit the sound barrier. On the other side of the barrier the plane's ride smoothed out again. That's a more appealing metaphor than thinking of myself as, say, a car that is simply over the hill, some ramshackle jalopy that gets more ramshackle with every pothole it encounters."

But even a jet plane eventually has to slow down again and return to earth.

One comes to understand that life is not a continuous ascent, or even a plateau. Time bears us up and then brings us back down.

The greater loss, some have thought, is not the eventual landing but the descent. Having experienced the fullness of one's flowering, one must bear the pruning process of aging. "Our youth dying in us," Montaigne suggested, is "really a harder death than the final dissolution of a languishing body, than the death of old age."[22] "How hard and painful are the last days of an aged man!" wrote the Egyptian philosopher poet Ptahhotep four and a half millennia ago.

> He grows weaker every day; his eyes become dim, his ears deaf; his strength fades; his heart knows peace no longer; his mouth falls silent and speaks no word. The power of his mind lessens and today he cannot remember what yesterday was like. All his bones hurt. Those things which not long ago were done with pleasure are painful now; and taste vanishes.

Old age, this ancient Egyptian concluded, "is the worst of misfortunes that can afflict a man."[23]

By the time the woodcutter comes to fell a tree thus pruned, to recall Gide's phrase, the severing of the trunk from the roots might not seem so great a blow.

DUST TO DUST

Aging is not so devastating for everyone, but ultimately we all come full cycle. Norman Cousins presents an arresting portrait of the elderly Pablo Casals. A frail old man shuffles to his instrument, and then immersed in his music he gathers strength and performs Bach with astounding vigor. But now even the vital Casals is vital no longer. Both he and the younger man who penned the account of Casals springing to life in his music have perished. While there are admirable models before us of living life to the full, it is not as though even one has shown us a way to escape our common destiny. Not one. In the words of the immortal Bard, "all that lives must die, / Passing through nature to eternity."[24]

The knowledge that death comes for us all is something toward which humanity must work its way, in both ontogenic and phylogenic terms. According to Choron, people in primitive societies understood the possibility but not the inevitability of death coming for any given person. Primitive man, he writes, "knows that he can die, but he does not know that he must die."[25] Students of the way the understanding of death evolves during childhood report something similar. At one stage—when they are roughly five to nine years of age—children conceive of death as a person, as someone "out there." As such, this "death person might be outwitted." (One thinks of the marvelous chess game against death in Ingmar Bergman's film *The Seventh Seal.)* "The clever or lucky person might not get caught."[26]

A death that *could* annihilate one but that one *might* elude is an altogether different threat from the humbling reality we eventually come to confront: that death is built into our nature, that it is part of the blueprint with which we are born, that it dwells, as it were, inside us. Medieval man, says Ariès, was "acutely conscious . . . that death was always present within him."[27] This notion of death within became vivid for me not very long ago when I visited the office of my dentist and friend, Harvey Levy, who advised me that it was time for a new set of X rays. Already thinking about mortality, I was struck by the image of myself grinning back off the film like the figure of death one finds in the paintings of the late Middle Ages. Another case of the obvious being nonetheless shocking: the figure we have learned to see as the menacing figure of death is there inside us all the time, simply camouflaged by our temporary cloak of corruptible flesh.

Death as an external enemy, as an affront, as something that imposes itself upon us. As though somehow it violates rather than fulfills nature. World cultures are replete with myths to explain how death entered the world—Adam and Eve's punishment for disobedience being only the best-known illustration—as though the natural order of things would be free of such hardship. Simone de Beauvoir wrote that "there is no such thing as a natural death," saying that for each person death represents "an unjustifiable violation." About this attitude, Malcolm Muggeridge conjures up an image of a demonstration "led by Madame de Beauvoir, and all the demonstrators chanting in unison: 'Death out! Death out!' "[28]

Something so marvelous as oneself should go on forever, we feel in our narcissistic hearts. But the oak tree is also marvelous, yet it too eventually returns to decompose on the forest floor. Before the modern era in Europe, people kept before them images of dead and decomposing human bodies, says Ariès, to maintain an "awareness of the failure to which each human life is condemned."[29]

Ashes to ashes, dust to dust—these phrases describe a cycle, the beginning and end points of the human life cycle.

TEMPORARY EMPIRES

We are but temporary aggregations of matter and energy. Not the gods we might wish to think ourselves.

Our temporariness we have in common. The dying frequently realize, and seek to remind us, that their situation and ours are not so different. Finitude is finitude. Be mindful of our place in the great scheme of things.

Montaigne wrote:

> Aristotle tells us that there are certain little beasts upon the banks of the river Hypanis, that never live above a day: they which die at eight of the clock in the morning, die in their youth, and those that die at five in the evening, in their decrepitude: which of us would not laugh to see this moment of continuance put into the consideration of weal or woe? The most and the least, of ours, in comparison with eternity, or yet with the duration of mountains, rivers, stars, trees and even of some animals, is no less ridiculous.[30]

We'd like to think our personal empires permanent, but nothing is ours to keep. "Nothing can ever take that away from you," said the mother of the woman awarded the master's degree; but the woman, outliving her capacity to use her education, learned otherwise.[31] Even for the healthy and the fortunate, it is all ours only on loan.

In my book *Fool's Gold* I wrote a section called "Indian Giver." It concerns different cultural attitudes toward property, contrasting the Native American's notion of special items as gifts that must be kept moving from one person to another with the European sense of possession. It concludes with reflections on how our "White Man Keeper" attitudes conflict with some fundamental truths about the nature of human life. "Life is a gift that is not ours to keep. All we can do is pass that gift along in our tribe, which alone endures. The Lord giveth and the Lord taketh away. There's the archetypal Indian giver."[32]

Our tribe alone endures. As marvelous as may be the individual oak tree, or the individual human being, the greater miracle lies in a whole that far transcends the individual and ephemeral parts.

Nothing Much

It was appalling to me how lovely was the weather in the Twin Cities on October third and fourth, 1967. A crystal blue Minnesota sky, with warm autumnal sun. There should have been lowering thunderclouds, turbulent winds, rumbling earthquakes, as in *Ben Hur* when Jesus expired on the cross. Some kind of dark omen, at least, some shudder of the cosmos, for on the early hours of the third my father strained and rasped for his final breaths, and on the fourth his body was laid into the earth. But the weather was perfect, adding a kind of insult to the grave injury of my loss. On the evening of the fourth, when Walter Cronkite wrapped up his newscast with his usual "That's the way it is," I felt like crying out, "That's not the way it is at all! You missed the banner-headline story of the day."

How could the departure forever of a man like my father go so unnoted by both universe and nation? There can be pain in recognizing how trifling one is in the great scheme of things.

Tethered to a dying animal. Watching my father, with whom I strongly identified, come to the end of his short life was one powerful message about my standing in the big picture. The affliction of my own body a couple of decades later has been another. I have found it difficult, as an ill man, to be honest and self-important at the same time. In a cover story in *Newsweek* about the physicist

Stephen Hawking—whose brilliant mind is confined to a disease-ravaged, largely paralyzed, wheelchair-bound body—his former wife is quoted as saying that her role in Hawking's life had become limited to reminding him that he is not God. My reaction upon reading that was, How on earth could someone in his deteriorating condition possibly need such reminding?

Yet the need to be reminded how insignificant any one of us is in the big picture is not so terribly rare. The grotesquely inflated narcissism of some of the tyrants of our time I find hideous. But as repugnant as I find Saddam Hussein's plastering his image on every wall in Iraq, or Ferdinand Marcos's project to have a one-man Rushmore of himself made of a mountain of a rock in the Philippines, there is a part of me that understands this desire to make the world as full of oneself as is one's own experience.

"I couldn't bear it," writes Betty Rollin of the disturbing normality of the streets in the wake of her devastation by breast cancer. She couldn't bear "that everything outside had remained exactly the same: . . . the Italian vegetable and fruit market with the same over-priced raspberries, the same swirl of people, moving down and up the street with the same unnerving briskness. And there, too, was the grotesquely pretty, midday sunshine."[33] Similarly, Diane Cole says, in her account of her hours as a hostage, threatened with sudden death by the Hanafi Muslims that had seized her office building: "The realization that the world would continue without me as it had before me was terrifying and humbling."[34]

Humbling. This opens a window looking out beyond the pain. For those completely trapped by the wounds and the compensation of the narcissistic undertaking—for the Hitlers and Saddam Husseins among us—being humbled can only be experienced as being humiliated. But for the rest of us, being humbled can represent a kind of liberation.

The election of Bill Clinton showed me that my illness had brought me a kind of freedom I didn't used to have. A whole cadre of people from my generation and my cultural tribe will be coming to power, I thought, and I will not be among them. Had this happened a few years before, being left out of the game like that would have bothered me. But now, it was perfectly fine. If the job got done well, it didn't matter whether or not I was in on the action. I don't matter so terribly much, I noted to myself, and it doesn't matter that I don't matter.

I thought of Aesop's fable about the flea who goes to great lengths to get the attention of an elephant and asks if it is all right with the great beast if he—the flea—moves from one ear to another. When he finally gets the elephant to hear his question, the elephant responds that he wasn't aware that the flea was there in the first place. The point of the story, as I have always heard it, is the foolishness of the flea in overestimating his importance. When I thought of the story now, however, it occurred to me that it might have been quite freeing for the flea to realize that something so insignificant as he did not have to worry so much about the elephant.

"When comes to the end," wrote Father Leclerq, ". . . a man's life is nothing much." Is this an expression of despair? The book from which this quote is drawn is described by Tournier as speaking "of the joy of growing old."[35]

Not long before his death, Thomas Wolfe wrote a letter to his editor, Maxwell Perkins, from his sickbed. In it, Wolfe moves from what had been his regret about "all the work I had not done . . . all the work I had to do" to describe a very different spiritual place at which he had arrived. "I know that I am just a grain of dust," Wolfe confides. Does this new knowledge devastate the dying man? As a result of his having come to see that he is but a grain of dust, he continues, "I feel as if a great window has been opened on life I did not know about before—and if I come through this, I hope to God I am a better man, and in some strange way I can't explain, I know I am a deeper and wiser one."[36]

PART II

Rising from
the Ashes

CHAPTER 5

Coming to Terms

On the Possibility and Value of Acceptance

UNTIMELY LOSS

I was supposed to be working on this book, but my energy just wasn't there. I had put on my old "Zorba the Greek" record, and tried dancing my way back into vigor ("Did you say, 'Dance!' "), but that just tired me further. "Why do the young die?" Zorba asks Alan Bates, who couldn't tell him. "If your books don't tell you that, what the hell do they tell you?" I heard this again in my mind as I trudged upstairs to lie down for a while. "They tell me," replies Bates's character, "of the agony of men who could not answer questions like yours." I sure as hell wanted my book to tell about more than that kind of agony.

What seemed most difficult for me to accept was how premature my debilitation was. Frequently, I felt like an old man, I moved like an old man. And I was tired of railing like Lear against the elements.

A knock on the door roused me from my rest. It was a new

neighbor of ours, coming over to introduce himself. I had heard sounds of someone working on the grounds next door and had intended to go over myself if I felt up to it. Our family is the only year-round inhabitant in our part of the ridge, the others being weekenders from the city, two-plus hours away, so meeting neighbors must be accomplished when the opportunity knocks. But I hadn't been able to rouse myself to go over there, and here was the neighbor doing the knocking.

His name was Bob Volger, and it turned out we could hardly have asked for a better neighbor: friendly, bright, interesting. Volger still stood straight, with not much hair on top but with humor in his eyes. But I couldn't say that meeting him on this particular occasion was a pleasure. I could not help contrast his vivaciousness with my own lethargy. Witnessing the vitality of others had often been disheartening before. But the contrast with Volger was especially hard to accept, because this gentleman was *thirty years older than I.* That we seemed to have switched roles was hard to bear.

Once again, the world has violated some kind of contract. A high-energy guy like me should have become a Volger-like septuagenarian; certainly in my forties I should have been a veritable dynamo. It wasn't time for me to be feeble.

The week before, I had gone to visit my mother to help prepare her place for winter. I did manage to accomplish my mission, more or less, but our time together was really more about her taking care of me than vice versa. As I lay on the rug, exhausted after my not-so-great labors, she prepared me a nourishing meal and plied me with the verbal equivalent of chicken soup as well. It was like being a kid again, and in that way comforting. But since it was forty years later, and it was I now in the prime of life and she elderly, it was also a reversal of the proper roles that part of me could not accept, just as I inwardly protested the contrast between my elderly neighbor's vivacity and my own frailty.

We have expectations about how things are supposed to pro-gress—with plenty of time to become accustomed to our finitude, plenty of time after one gets to the top of the hill to get used to being over the hill. These expectations function like what I called "bargains with the world." With respect to mortality, for example, Feifel speaks of "the private arrangements" we make with death. Most prominent among these private arrangements, he writes, concerns an orderliness in Death's progress through the genera-tions. "Most people anticipate that the oldest of their important people will be the first to die." The belief in such orderliness gives some comfort. "The fact that Death calls the person 'first in line' shows that it is playing the game fairly, faithful to the unwritten rules. The death of an old person can help to support the survivor's belief that a kind of rationality prevails. One's own turn will not be coming up for a while."[1] There's supposed to be an order. The flow of powers is supposed to follow the rules. It should have been Volger's turn to be feeble, not mine.

I had been brought up not to swallow injustice. Now the unfair-ness of the switch in vitality between Volger's generation and mine was stuck in my throat. Yet as we walked around my hillside orchard, I felt some piece of my attitude ready to drop off like some fruit that had at last ripened. Protesting whatever is unfair—any violation of the rules—had served me well through most of my life, as a social critic and political actor in the world, for example. But in this instance, protest wasn't about to change anything but would only poison me and wear me down. Give it up, I told myself. This is where I am, so be there. I spoke to myself in Hamlet's words: "If it be now, 'tis not to come; if it be not to come, it will be now; if it be not now, yet it will come."[2] The readiness, as Hamlet said, is all.

I began to relax into enjoying getting acquainted with Volger. As he left and walked up the hill of our driveway with the stride of someone my age, I at first began to bring on the pain of saying to myself, "why can't I do that?" Stopping myself, I leaned back in

my mind and made a shift. Like some retired athlete who still loves
the game from the sidelines, I found I took real pleasure in the
thought, "Isn't it neat that a guy his age is still so full of life?"

KISSING THE FROG

For the first time, I started to be able to say to myself, "If this is the
hand I have to play from here on out, so be it. I'll make the best of
it." Not resignation, exactly, since I continued to be resolved to
persist in seeking full health by whatever means I could discover.
But some kind of acceptance, some sense—previously lacking—
that even if nothing improved, it would be okay. Not the fate I
wanted, but, if it was mine, I would take it.

The interesting part was that concurrent with this acceptance, I
began to feel better. It was not clear that the symptoms had less-
ened, but I had a sense that there was more of me living there. My
soul seemed to have seeped back into me.

Did the shift toward acceptance *cause* the improvement in how I
felt? I don't know. As I have often remarked with disgruntlement,
life is a very poorly controlled experiment. That was even more
than usually true in this, what with the spate of elixers and remedies
and concoctions I was also trying out at that time. Which *hoc* is
post which? I cannot rule out the possibility that the causality oper-
ated in the other direction: that my capacity to accept emerged at
this time because a shift in my underlying physiology simply made
my situation more acceptable.

While acknowledging that possibility, however, I chose to con-
centrate on the hypothesis that the feeling of *acceptance* conjured up
some kind of healing power. For years I had fought my plight with
an increasing sense of desperation at being stuck with the entirely
intolerable, and where had it gotten me? I had tried to remove this
card from my hand, to expel it like some ugly Old Maid, and it

stayed stuck and, if anything, had grown uglier. Maybe coming to accept the hand I'd been dealt was like the princess kissing the frog in the fairy tale. She discovers how the frog can be transformed into a prince only when she is able to look beyond the frog's ugliness and ineligibility as her suitor.

NEVER SAY DIE

Such acceptance comes easily to none of us. It also goes against the grain of our cultural values.

I am, or at least I was in an earlier incarnation, a football fan. The professional football player is one of the most conspicuous embodiments of our society's image of manly virtue. And, as the tens of millions of people who weekly watch football games can attest, the football player does not accept defeat—even inevitable defeat—so long as the clock still gives him one second of time.

That is why the last two minutes of playing time regularly take an eternity. Even if a team is hopelessly behind, it is expected to do everything in its power to delay the inevitable, to pretend that another outcome is possible. (In our culture of competition, the master who tips over his king early in the match to signal his concession of the defeat that has become visible to his expert eye is an alien figure.) Time-outs are used, sideline pass patterns are run, as if by sheer willpower the obstinate team might score four unanswered touchdowns in the last couple minutes. Never say die! That's supposed to be a man's attitude.

That approach—carried to an extreme—can ruin the dramatic flow of a football game. But how does it affect the drama of one's life?

Evidence suggests that a fighting spirit can have substantial adaptive value. Apparently, a good deal of the decline associated with the aging process is a function of lifestyle, and those who fight to maintain their vitality enjoy considerable success. To cite just one example, only about one-third of the diminution, usually seen in our society, of a person's aerobic capacity appears to be due to the natural aging process, while the other two-thirds of the deterioration is caused by inactivity.

The fighting spirit can help also with illness. Cousins and Siegel both cite studies indicating that certain kinds of struggle and even negativity directed against one's illness are correlated with longer survival for patients with cancer. Among women with metastatic breast cancer, "long-term survivors had higher scores for negative emotional expression than did short-term survivors." The long-term survivors seemed, to their oncologists, "significantly less 'well adjusted' to their illnesses" than the short-term survivors.[3]

The meaning of this finding, however, is not self-evident. Is it helpful to *be* more negative or is the issue that it is not constructive to suppress those negative feelings one has? The long-term survivors "expressed their emotions freely"[4]: perhaps it is this freedom rather than the negativity that correlates with not succumbing to the disease. (How do patients with a suppression-free attitude of positive acceptance fare?) When doctors rate "well adjustedness," perhaps what they are rating is how little the patients compel those around them to confront the patients' experience of pain and fear and grief.

In another study, conducted in London, more than three times as many of those cancer patients who had a "fighting spirit" survived ten years as did those with "stoic acceptance" or with feelings of helplessness or hopelessness.[5] But again, there is room to wonder how clearly these dichotomies present our choices. Are hopelessness and helplessness the only alternatives to perpetual protest and resistance? Is there some kind of acceptance that is healthier than the stoic variety?

I make no pretense to knowing the answers to these questions I am posing. I do know my own "fighting spirit" took a toll. Peace is part of health. More and more, my goal became to achieve a state of mind that combined a determination to work for health with an acceptance of ongoing illness. Struggle in the midst of peace.

THE KNEE-HIGH MAN

There is a story I have long liked from African-American folklore: it is called "The Knee-High Man." In it, this little fellow is ambitious to become big, and so he goes around asking for advice from the various big folks in his neighborhood. These include a cow, a horse, and the like. Each one offers the same basic advice: do just what I do, and you will become large like I am. The horse, for example, counsels the knee-high man to eat lots and lots of oats and go running around in the fields, and assures him that as a result he will become as big as a horse. (After all, it worked for the horse.) But all the knee-high man gets from his emulation of the ways of the horse is a bellyache from the oats and exhaustion from the running around.

The knee-high man's story has come to my mind occasionally as I've read some of the treatises on overcoming illness written by those I call the "gung-hoers," those from the you-can-prevail, you-can-regain-all-you've-lost, you-can-be-happy school of thought. All these authors seem to think that the path they have blazed in their own lives lies available for anyone with the good sense and good character to choose to follow them. Frequently, I have felt like saying to the author: that path may get you out from where you were, but it doesn't seem to lead out from where I am.

That experience has impressed on me the importance of bringing a certain amount of humility to how we approach another person's suffering. It is hard to know just what someone else is having to contend with, or what choices are really available in the place they find themselves. This applies also to one extolling the value of "acceptance." I feel compelled to acknowledge that some forms of suffering, some losses, are a good deal easier to accept than others. There is illness, which takes many forms, as does aging. There is death, which can take away from us those whom we cherish and will eventually take us as well. There is the loss of vitality, and of various capabilities. And there is pain and discomfort—physical and mental—whose variety in degree and kind is as abundant as the wildflowers in a springtime meadow.

In his years as a teacher of transcendental meditation, my friend Reuel Young would explain TM's overall beneficial effect on one's well-being by saying, "It is hard to feel bad when you're feeling good." But many people in the grip of illness must confront the other side of that coin: it's hard to feel good when you are feeling bad.

"For there was never yet a philosopher who could endure the toothache patiently." Thus read the inscription on a greeting card send by a friend to Herbert Howe, author of *Do Not Go Gentle,* when that young man was in the throes of his battle with cancer. Some of the dying come to peace with their situation. But one of the chief impediments to this acceptance, evidently, is having to contend with serious pain. In "Living Until Death," Raymond Carey reports on the correlates with "emotional adjustment" to the process of one's own dying, and lists most saliently among these that "the more discomfort an individual suffered, the less able he was to maintain a high level of emotional adjustment."[6] If you are hard-pressed to bear the present moment, you'll apparently have more difficulty in accepting that the future you've anticipated has been taken away.

GO WITH THE FLOW

I couldn't tell if I had stumbled onto some wisdom or if it was just a piece of sophistry.

At a certain point in my illness, I decided to stop frustrating myself by contrasting how I felt with how I *ought* to feel; I told myself that feeling sick is just another way of being. At one level, I recognized, being ill is worse than being healthy. But at times I thought I had glimpses of a deeper level where one state is equivalent to another.

Did this amount to some kind of nihilism in which nothing matters? Was it mere sophistry? Or was I seeing something real?

As I found my way into that space, I felt more full with my crippled aliveness, and hence more satisfied with my experience than when I was seeking a kind of experience that didn't appear on my menu.

Whatever the experience, don't fight it—let it fill you and flow on through. When my cat Jason was killed, my grief was spontaneous and unhindered. It flowed through me like a flash flood. I cried cleanly and unashamedly—even with my daughter, Terra, present—as I gathered up Jason's body and buried him. There was for me something remarkable in the experience of my unobstructed grieving. Even while my grief was full upon me, even as I uncharacteristically sobbed, in some fundamental way *it didn't hurt*. It was a rich and alive experience, and it had a beginning and an end. When I was done crying, I was done. Like the rapid clearing after a thunderstorm, my life went on to other things. I still miss Jason, and can still contact my love for him, but dealing with his death was not a "negative" experience for me.

In *The Courage to Grieve*, Judy Tatelbaum writes that "confronting grief rather than avoiding it shortens the duration of the experience."[7] If that is the case, if so simple a procedure as letting the feelings happen is the way to healing, why do so many of us, so much of the time, resist our experience? With respect to grief, Ariès writes that Western societies of the past century and more have applied "a merciless coercion" to impose "the suppression of mourning."[8] Society, in Ariès' view, fears the expression of feelings whose intensity is too great—and many of us fear it for ourselves as well. I have known one widow who bore the great burden of her grief with considerable stoicism, saying that she feared that if she allowed herself to begin crying, she would never be able to stop. She had probably been taught, in a variety of implicit ways, that our emotional processes are not to be trusted, that we cannot rely upon our organism to take care of itself. Perhaps as a consequence of her fear of letting the grief flow, the grief lay upon her like a dark cloud of depression.

We fear also the experience of our pain. That fear has certainly been a major inhibition for me: it has often seemed that suffering might be more than I could bear if I allowed myself to experience it fully. So I have worked to resist it. But then there was my experience of mourning Jason the cat. When I didn't resist the pain and sadness, the pain seemed to be transformed into something much more endurable.

Pain would therefore seem to be a kind of limiting case for testing the go-with-the-flow strategy. In this perspective, it is especially interesting to consider the report by Stanislav Grof and Joan Halifax—in *The Human Encounter with Death*—from their work with dying patients. Providing dying cancer patients with a supportive human environment and with psychedelic substances, they explored what could be done for the terminally ill to make the final part of their lives a more meaningful and positive experience. How pain might be dealt with was an area of particular interest for their study.

The best way to deal with pain, they found, was by "focusing and concentrating on the pain with an accepting attitude." They concede that this posture toward the pain would appear to be "the exact opposite" of what we would expect to bring relief from an intolerable burden of pain. And, indeed, the first consequence of fully letting the pain in would seem to confirm one's inclination to resist and reject the pain: what happens first is "a temporary amplification of the unpleasant sensations to the point that the individual briefly reaches his or her experiential limit of pain." But then one finds one is able to "transcend" it: "paradoxically, accepting pain, yielding to it, 'going into it and with it' can make it possible to move experientially beyond pain altogether." Yielding to the impulse to reject unpleasant, but unavoidable, experience is an exercise in futility. "The least useful approach to pain," they report, "seems to be to let it occupy the center of awareness while at the same time resisting it and fighting against it."[9] Even with the intense pain of cancer in its terminal stages, it appears, the best way of navigating one's experience is to align oneself with the river's current.

The impulse to fight the river is entirely understandable, because we wouldn't choose as our destination where the river is taking us. But what does it profit us to put ourselves in opposition to the nature of things? This does not mean we must be altogether passive in the face of the forces that buffet us. In his discussion of aging, Paul Tournier seems to call for an approach that combines fundamental acceptance of one's fate with the possibility of a kind of control. Tournier calls for "a profound submission to the laws of nature." By this, he does not mean "capitulating to natural scourges": we can work to make our trip down the river more comfortable. But that it is in the nature of things that we will be swept along the river—to that fundamental destiny he counsels us to submit. Francis Bacon's famous statement, at the outset of the scientific era—"One commands Nature only by obeying her"—Tournier recasts to illuminate the experience of aging, saying that "in the same way, one commands old age only by obeying it."[10]

CHOICES

"You can't lose a lot of sleep," says the prominent journalist dying of AIDS, "being bitter because you're one of the ones suffering."[11] Of course, taken on the face of it, that statement is false: one *can* get all agitated and bitter about one's fate. What he means, one may suppose, is that such bitterness serves no good purpose, that it only compounds one's suffering.

It is important to recognize that one does have choices.

"Someone once lauded to [Freud] Franz Rosenzweig's courageous tolerance of his total paralysis, and Freud responded, 'What else can he do?' "[12] Freud seems to have begrudged Rosenzweig the praise, for surely Freud had ample imagination to answer his own rhetorical question. If Rosenzweig had come to terms with his unfortunate condition, he had accomplished no small feat.

In Berman's fine collection *The Courage to Grow Old,* one line struck me as running like a refrain through the various anthologized statements. Berman had invited a variety of prominent older Americans to describe their experience of aging, and several of the respondents, quite independently, had employed the same quotation to articulate a central part of the state of mind they had achieved as they moved through the final stages of their lives: "I accept the universe." The story behind that quotation, evidently, is that a woman once made that declaration within the hearing of Ralph Waldo Emerson. Emerson is said to have retorted, "She had better."

Emerson's response seems both flippant and obtuse. Sure, one might say, "One has no choice but to accept the universe" in the same sense that one "can't" be bitter about one's suffering. But that sense obscures the profound spiritual challenge one faces in accepting without bitterness what the universe has dealt one.

From some people whom I love, the heartfelt declaration "I accept the universe" would make me weep with relief on their behalf.

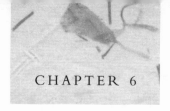

CHAPTER 6

The Virtues of Our Necessities

On Possibilities of Gaining from Our Adversities

TREASURE IN THE FIELDS

An old farmer, when he was dying, called his somewhat shiftless sons to his bedside. He told them that he was leaving them a treasure, but all he would tell them about its location was that it was buried somewhere in the fields. After the father's death, the sons frantically dug up the fields searching for their inheritance. Finding nothing, they decided that, inasmuch as the fields were all dug up anyway, they might as well plant some crops. The resulting harvest put them in good stead for the coming year. The next spring they again searched all over for the buried treasure of which their father had spoken on his deathbed. Again their search was fruitless, and again, as an afterthought, they planted crops into the overturned soil. And so it went for a few years until, having developed the habits of good farmers and grown prosperous from their labors, they forgot all about their dreams of easy riches.

That's a fable by Aesop. I've always liked it, but my efforts to restore my health brought new meaning to it for me. The treasure

I've sought was some kind of cure; the digging has been the healing work I did on my body. I did acupuncture and got my meridians balanced; I got rolfed and got my body straighter and more balanced; I overhauled my diet so that I waste hardly a calorie on food that is not nourishing; I tuned into the benefits of stopping eating when the body has had enough, forgoing that last 25 percent of the meal that, as the saying goes, feeds one's doctor; the bellows of my cranial-sacral rhythm were smoothened; I studied and adopted the practices for good and regular sleep.

That all this did not bring a cure was not a trivial shortcoming of this multidimensional regimen. The fact that each practitioner was satisfied, at the end of our work together, that he or she said that I had made great progress, I could, I suppose, have dismissed with allusion to that old line "The operation was a success but the patient died." But I chose to look at a more positive aspect of the picture. That's where Aesop came in. Necessity taught me how to tend the needs of my body. I learned to cultivate the habits of healthful living. Ultimately, I thought, like the sons in the fable, my efforts will prove to sustain me.

In youth, and in the boisterous bloom of health, we are apt to take our bodies for granted. Identifying with our perhaps ungrounded will, with our many unwise wants, we may treat the totality of our organism as but a convenient instrument for our gratification. If a food tastes good in the mouth, down it goes. If there are exciting doings around, to hell with sleep. One's body can be like a partner a thoughtless person uses for pleasure in the evening and fails to respect in the morning.

A person's native vigor can obscure the ongoing erosion of his or her underlying resources, the way farmers in America's fertile prairies can keep going strong while foot after foot of the abundant topsoil inherited from nature washes off their fields into rivers and ultimately out to sea.

When our resources are in short supply, we are led to learn the skills of resource management. We learn what depletes and we learn what replenishes, and we shift our practices accordingly or we suffer ever more serious breakdowns of our organismic economy. When the body can no longer be taken for granted, we are encouraged to build a different kind of relationship with it. Instead of perceiving it as a date that we might, in our callousness and callowness, treat as an object, we discover the need to foster a deeper partnership, a bond with give-and-take and mutual respect. As a consequence of the experience of illness, Brody writes, "I may come to listen more sympathetically to my body, to see it as a source of values that legitimately should play a role in how I live my life, and not simply as having value only when it carries out the wishes of other aspects of the self."[1]

Two commentators on illness that I came across employ the image of marriage. "The chronic wounds of illness," Levitt and Guralnick write in *You Can Make It Back*, "are married to our flesh. Like a clinging wife or husband, the wound that occupies our life won't let us be alone. . . . All future plans, all rendezvous, all leaves of absence must include our wound."[2] When Arnold Beisser, the young doctor and player struck down by polio, writes, "I find that my relationship with my disability is similar to a marriage," his sounds like a somewhat happier marriage than the "petulant and jealous" spouse in the image from Levitt and Guralnick. "We have an agreement, my disability and I," Beisser writes. "It requires that I take care of it, and it will allow me to do what I want. . . . It is not an altogether unfriendly relationship. Sometimes it is even a love relationship."[3]

Another image Beisser uses for the relationship between himself and the disability afflicting his body is the one between a teacher and a student. "My disability has taught me much, and continues to do so. It teaches me about limitations and about the hazards of pride and vanity."[4]

My own image from Aesop is similar: illness has been my

teacher, helping me learn the ways of health. In my reading, I have discovered that two giants of American cultural history of the nineteenth century made observations along the same lines. One of the outstanding men of American medicine, William Osler, said that the chronically ill learn to live a long life.[5] And that great jurist Oliver Wendell Holmes said that the best way to ensure a long, productive life is to "have a chronic disease and take care of it."[6]

The laboratory tests results were back, and while it remained still unclear what ailed me, evidence was accumulating that my digging in the field was producing its own kind of treasure.

Three of my four grandparents died of coronary and hypertensive diseases, and so I looked with particular interest at the signs of where I might be on that slippery slope. If one can believe the current medical understanding of the precursors of coronary disease, my numbers were a good crop. Cholesterol level at 156, a Cholesterol/HDL ratio (at 2.83) one would choose if one could, and a level of iron in the blood toward the low end of normal. Mark Twain may have wanted to preserve some vices so he'd have something to throw overboard in an emergency, but I prefer the tack of avoiding the emergencies in the first place.

In early years, I displayed the family's knack for converting stress into an elevation of blood pressure. When I went for my army physical in 1968, my numbers escalated into the range where medication would have been called for had my old football back problem not earned me a 1-Y classification (thus helping my pressure return to a fairly normal 125/85). When my first marriage was breaking up, my numbers again crossed the threshold above normal. Now, as my body taught me in a number of palpable ways that stress takes a toll, I learned to live more gently. As a result, I think, of my newfound appreciation of life in the slow lane, my numbers routinely came in at 110/70. Hardly like a Schmookler.

It has been an expensive education in its way, I thought, but God willing it will prove worth it.

MAKING THE BEST OF IT

Low cholesterol numbers, of course, did not entirely compensate for all the other diminutions that had occurred in me. Losses such as those described in chapter 2, "Living Posthumously," have to be mourned—and then they have to be adapted to.

I wondered, who am I if I'm no longer the same achiever I was? Standing convicted in my own mind of being now a lesser being, could I manage to acquit myself by pleading diminished capacity? I had always been a high-energy person. I'd taken pride in my tirelessness. But the energy was depleted now, and although I could at times reach down for it, I seemed to pay a high price for maintaining that old identity. In my work, I always took on big questions and tried to surround them single-handedly, to storm them by sheer force of irresistible effort. If this is no longer a feasible—or even appealing—way to proceed, I asked myself, how do I continue to work as a creative person?

As I wrote what was eventually published as *Fool's Gold: The Fate of Values in a World of Goods,* I discovered a new way of working. In the stead of my old monumental style of painting panoramas, I adopted more of a Zen brushstroke technique. A few aptly executed lines can suggest a great deal of a landscape that the resonances in the imagination of the reader can flesh out. This more restrained style not only suited better my present capacities and the quality of my energy, it also had certain charms of its own. I might not have come to it had my vigor maintained, but I was not sure I regret the shift.

While exploring the subject of aging, I asked my friend Ken Mayers—roughly a decade my senior, and growing older well—for his thoughts on the subject, based on his own experience. In reply, he told the following joke. A new young bull on the farm was being shown around the place by the old bull. From the top of the hill, they spied a herd of cows. "Those cows," said the old bull, "are for us to service." "Wow!" responded the young bull, "I've got a great idea: let's run down there and hump one of those cows." "I've got a better idea," countered the old bull. "Let's *walk* down there and hump them all."

Part of adapting to the scarcities that come with aging, or with illness, is to manage better what resources we have. The work can assume a different pace and spirit from what characterized the efforts of one's more abundant and profligate youth. Robert J. Lifton, citing the work of Elliot Jacques on changes in the work of artists and musicians in middle age, speaks of a "sculpted" quality in the work of older artists, the fruit of a mode of work that is "slower, more careful and painstaking," in contrast with the more "intense" and "spontaneous" quality of work done earlier in life.[7]

The natural slowing down that comes with the passage of years is not, of course, the only—and certainly not the worst—change with which a person may have to contend. How does one find a way, in the face of genuine disability, to preserve what is essential in one's identity as a productive person, as one who creates something of value out of one's skills and, perhaps, out of one's very being?

This is a problem that Janet Maurer and Patricia Strasberg explore in their book *Building a New Dream*. An architect with Parkinson's disease struggled to continue to be productive. When he could not hold a pencil steadily enough to draw up the blueprints, he mastered a computer program that enabled him to do the blueprints. When his disability progressed to the point that he was incapable of using the computer, he retired, with the result that he felt useless and became dejected. He then found a way to make a comeback. "He designed in his head and used a draftsman to have it put on paper. After that, Joe spoke to the town board and was invited to sit on the architectural planning committee. He also volunteered to help other family members and friends design bathrooms or porches on their homes."[8]

Illness can strip a person of his or her abilities, leaving only bits and pieces of the edifice that had been there before. But often the pieces that remain include the essential core of the structure, and a way can be found to preserve the soul of one's old work. To a carpenter disabled from working the hours and lifting the materials of his former work life, Maurer and Strasberg counsel: "You can also train or supervise. Your knowledge is in your head and in your mind's eye." Though your hands are disabled, your creativity and knowledge are intact.[9]

If mind and soul remain unimpaired, even frailties of the body that seem to threaten the continuation of one's world can often be transcended. John McLeish describes how the great painter Auguste Renoir overcame the impediment of crippling arthritis. Stricken in his early fifties, Renoir found his hands becoming ever more twisted, until at last he could not squeeze his own paints onto his palette and could not hold a brush save by having the brush affixed to "an apparatus attached to his rigid fingers and wrist." Nevertheless, writes McLeish, he continued to paint great works until his death.

> Nothing exhausted his great talent—in fact it was inexhaustible, because it was not a bank deposit to be drawn on but an underground river constantly fed by Renoir's own marvellous love of life, sensitivity to colour, and openness to the continuous wonder of human experience.[10]

What we are left with often can seem most paltry and unsatisfactory. Renoir's affliction could have been worse: he did not, after all, become blind. But what about poor Beethoven, for whom there was no apparatus that could be strapped to him to substitute for his vanished capacity? Like the man discussed earlier who developed the capacity to "hallucinate" fragrances he could no longer sense, Beethoven found ways to fill in with his imagination what he could no longer directly hear. A touching scene is described by Ludwig Carmolini in his account of his last visit with Beethoven. Beethoven asked his friend and student to sing, confessing that as he can hear nothing he only wants to *see* him sing. "When I finished, Beethoven motioned me near to him, pressed my hand cordially, and said, 'From your breathing I can see that you sing correctly, and in your eyes I have read that you feel what you sing. It has been a great pleasure for me.' "[11]

Perhaps Beethoven's expression of pleasure was only a polite gesture, but I prefer to think of the great composer having achieved the further greatness of in fact getting pleasure from the signs, without being able to apprehend the full resonant substance, of what had been his greatest joy.

Like trees on a cliff face that somehow manage to extend their roots into the slightest cracks in the rocks to draw their sustenance, some human beings display an inspiring capacity to find a niche of pleasure under the most inhospitable of conditions. Shortly before her death from cancer, one woman still appeared to be in good spirits, say Stanislav Grof and Joan Halifax. "Although the passage through her stomach was now totally obstructed and she could not swallow anything," they write, this woman still "insisted that she be served all the meals that others were eating. . . . She chewed the food slowly, savored its taste, and then spat it out into a bucket."[12]

NEW ME

"A refusal to bury the dead." Unto this is what Robert Kastenbaum likens holding desperately to a former version of the self, which the passage of time has taken away. Even without illness, the years will compel one to replace "who-I-have-been" with who-I-am-still-becoming." A harmonious transition is possible, says Kastenbaum. But, often in midlife, a failure to make this transition results in what he calls a "developmental death"—a refusal to bury the dead, meaning those parts of the former self that are withered or gone. Or, alternatively, "The person 'buries the dead,' and crawls into the grave along with the corpse."[13] The person, that is, lives posthumously in the worst sense—not really living. Not accepting as a real life what is still available, such a person says to himself, as Kastenbaum puts it, "That part of my life is over, and so I am over, too."[14]

With the losses that illness can impose, it can be especially difficult to find in the "new me" that remains an acceptable identity. Difficult, but not impossible. "I've finally stopped competing with the late, great me," says a woman debilitated by chronic fatigue syndrome.[15] "Finally"—the word suggests the battering to which chronicity subjects one: old habits of thought die hard. "If you have the flu for a week or two," says another woman, "you have the luxury of feeling sorry for yourself, but with a chronic illness you've got to gain control of your reactions." That control requires the ability to redefine, to reconceive one's mission, to find new sources of meaning, ultimately to arrive at a new conception of oneself.

One man, in the process of rehabilitating from severe burn injuries, chose a new name for himself.[16] This is a rather blatant way of representing a transition in identity of a kind that many of us, in the course of our lifetimes, must achieve: I am no longer the person I was.

Sometimes, the new identity is constructed around the very wounds that obliterated the old. Lois Jaffe was a woman dying from leukemia who utilized her experience to help health professionals explore issues surrounding death and dying. Asked what problem she would face if doctors found a cure for leukemia, she replied ("after a long, breathless pause"): "I would have to find a new identity."[17]

A sculptress named Nancy Reid had a mastectomy. Living "in a culture where breasts are supposed to be young and blemish-free forever," she felt devastated. She felt "mutilated and sexless." Eventually, however, her struggle with her mutilation led to her most successful sculptures. Early pieces in the series were of tormented women, furious and screaming, with breasts coming out of odd places. As she continued to work publicly with her pain and loss, the series produced a sculpture "of a one-breasted woman holding her skirts out on each side the way little girls sometimes do. It's a proud and sexy figure defiantly called 'The Flirt.' . . . I did [the Flirt] when I realized that there's life, there's sexuality, after mastectomy."[18]

Change. It is part of the life process whether we choose for it to be or not. Whether we suffer the sudden catastrophic losses of illness or "only" the more seamless transformations of the life cycle, living our whole lives fully requires the capacity to make transitions from one stage of life, with its corresponding identity, to the next. This is a difficult challenge, and one that our culture does not greatly aid us in meeting.

Perhaps a cultural paradox is to be found here. No cultural system in human history has been so dedicated to change, so dynamic in its entire stance, as Western civilization. When it comes to the overall framework in which our lives are embedded—the landscape, the institutional systems—in modern Western societies it is true, as Marx put it, that "all that is solid melts into air." But when it comes to the changes that are part of the individual life process, a different attitude seems to be entrenched in our culture. When we look at Western culture "from the point of view of life stages,"

Grof and Halifax write, "we see that the time of major transitions from one stage in life to another is usually fraught with a negative value." Even birth, they observe, may be included, treated as it is in negative terms, as a medical problem. But their generalization, they say, "is certainly true for puberty, middle age, senescence, and, of course, dying."[19]

If there is a contradiction here, from what would it arise? Perhaps the attachment to change in the macrocosmic scale is a function of the Western infatuation with the notion of "progress"—ever onward and upward, eternal growth and improvement; whereas progress and improvement without end at the level of the individual human destiny is clearly at odds with the facts of our animal existence. Indeed, the quest for the ever-expanding empire of the larger human system may be, in part, an attempt to deny and to distract from the inescapable cycle of the human life.

Perhaps this is why traditional societies—which as a whole strive to maintain stability rather than foment continual revolution—provide meaningful rites of passage to assist their members in making the transition from the identity appropriate for one stage of life into that for the next; whereas, when we who live in a society in constant upheaval seek to find positive meaning in the transition from one stage of life to another, we discover that we are largely on our own.

LIFE IS NOT AN OLYMPIC EVENT

With a new identity come new values.

If I finally stop competing with the late, great me, it is because the old system of valuation continually makes me a loser. I have a choice. I can persist in my old ways of keeping score and continually experience failure. Or I can sever my attachment to that old scoring system.

The transformation of values is thus propelled by a strong motivation, and this transformation could thus be dismissed as mere rationalization—like the king in the story who shoots an arrow at a wall and then has his men draw a target around wherever it sticks. But the old system of values was not necessarily the last word in human wisdom. Formed early in life in response to an environment that was doubtless less than ideal, one's original way of construing life is likely to be a source of problems as well as a solution to them. The breakdown of that orientation under the onslaught of misfortune, which one experiences initially as unwelcome and painful, can thus provide an important opportunity for spiritual advance.

Wisdom through suffering is an idea with an ancient pedigree.

I always had a heroic approach to life. Outstanding achievement was, from early on, my principal strategy for feeling good about myself. It is easy to see how it was encouraged in my family. In large measure, it worked. The problem with that solution is that it solidifies a precariousness about one's self-acceptance. Being okay must continually be earned. One is always dependent on one's capacity to *do;* simply *being* who one is is insufficient to yield one peace of mind. If some kind of winning is required, always lurking in the shadow is the role of the loser.

The emerging inability to *do* as I used to drove me to regard the human condition somewhat differently. The "heroism" of "ordinary" people became visible to me. For some people, I started to grasp, just getting out of bed in the morning and seeing that the children get off to school all right is a great achievement. Taking pride in being "special" came to seem to be based on a very hollow perspective.

Some days I would get up and do "good" work. Other days it took a greater effort simply to get up and to cope with the demands of daily life. How important really, I asked myself, is the difference between these "achievements"?

Moira Griffin writes of a change in her experience with attending dance class:

> All those years when I would "demonstrate" an exercise or a dance move, trying not to look like I was loving it, trying not to look like I was showing off a bit. . . . Now I go to the back row, so as not to alarm other students, so as not to be stared at by them. There must be an easier way to learn that a talent is good luck and hard work, not some kind of superiority and hard work. Did I really deserve to be good then? Do I really deserve to be bad now? Oh, well. Just do it if you can do it, Griffin.[20]

Relinquishing pride, letting go of that quest for personal empire. This is a key lesson of that most profound of literary genres, tragic drama, where the hero becomes in some profound way larger when he lets go of false self-magnification. And it can be a consequence of those tragedies that befall us in our own lives.

Kavanaugh looks for "the key that unlocks serenity in the dying." He finds it in "that poverty of spirit almost all religious or spiritual leaders recommend for life." (For life, not just for death—for we are all among "the dying.") This poverty of spirit, writes Kavanaugh, "is an attitude of detachment from all that is not truly our own."[21]

So what is it that is truly our own? I think of that old Gestalt phrase, "being in the here and now."

Now is the only time there is. Faust, that prototypical empire-builder of our civilization, had it exactly wrong. In their bargain, Faust was to suffer damnation at that moment when he felt so in love with the "now" that he ceased to be oriented toward the next moment's coming. But in truth—a truth that illness and aging seem able to bring home to us—it is when we cannot live in the moment that we are damned.

One of the respondents to the *Sun*'s inquiry about aging, L. B.

Chase, identifies as one of the fruits or signs of his growing older that he no longer thinks of his experience as a prelude, leading "to something important." He goes on: "I realize now that there has been no prelude, just life itself, all along."[22]

No prelude, only now. As in the Zen story, the wise man—clinging to the side of the cliff—relishes his moment before annihilation and savors the wild strawberry he discovers growing within reach of his hand. This is a wisdom that some who are brought low by illness or are poised on the edge of the grave discover growing out of their adversity.

Just as "now" is found to be at the center of time, located between an irretrievable past and an unreachable future, so also is there a core part of the self that is more truly one's own. Beneath the peripheral layers that one may have learned to mistake for who one is, there are disclosed the more essential elements of one's being. Again, it is upon what from one viewpoint is a process of deterioration that a deeper awareness can be grounded; it is out of loss that we can gain in understanding.

In an article on menopause, potentially one of the more difficult losses in the cycle of a woman's life, Anne Schleider is quoted as saying that "the prettier a woman is in her youth, the more insecure she is" when she undergoes menopause. "When the looks start to go, she's not left with much." What is she left with when the peripheral layers that had been the source of value and identity are stripped away? "As I grew up, I thought all I was was a body and a face," says the television actress Rita Rifkin. "I thought that everything had to be perfect on the outside." Consequently, menopause at first plunged her into a state of hopelessness. But now, she says, she is finding out that what makes her feel like a "real woman" is "grabbing every second you can and living life to the fullest."[23] Not what one looks like from the outside, but what one experiences on the inside.

A movement of attention from the external to the internal,

from the superficial to the essential, from the periphery to the core.

That woman who, ravaged by cancer and chemotherapy, had been horror-struck by her own appearance and who had her husband remove all the mirrors from the walls of their house, eventually came to a deeper place. "Mirrors hold no terror now. . . . Visitors tell of an inner beauty reflected in recent smiles." Hers is a loss one would never choose. Yet what she gains in exchange for that loss is a treasure. "Instead of the indignity I feared, I now feel human love can deepen in nakedness, if pride disappears."[24]

Lois Jaffe, the woman who used her terminal leukemia as an opportunity to teach doctors about death and dying, writes that she always closed her seminars with a favorite passage from *The Velveteen Rabbit,* by Margery Williams Bianco. In it, the Skin Horse is explaining to the Rabbit about being "Real." Becoming Real, says the Skin Horse, "takes a long time."

> That's why it doesn't often happen to people who break easily, or have sharp edges, or who have to be carefully kept. Generally, by the time you are Real, most of your hair has been loved off, and your eyes drop out, and you get loose in the joints and very shabby. But these things don't matter at all, because once you are Real, you can't be ugly, except to people who don't understand.[25]

I can think of no loss more wrenching than the death of one's child. But even such a wound can be an opportunity for growth. Families struggling with such a loss tend to undergo a shift in their values. From focusing on "material wealth, status, and worldly goals of success and achievement," these families in the wake of the death of a child tend to move toward a new perspective in which "family, community, and spiritual" values are more central.

If we all grew up straight and tall, with our roots sunk deep into the sacred spring of human spiritual values, we would have no need of blows to awaken us, and all they would bring us would be the bruises. But, for most of us, disaster can serve as an opportunity, shaking down our flimsier structures and giving us a new chance to build from a solid foundation.

BRAVE NEW COSMOS

It had been a good week. My energy felt clear—maybe not as strong as I wished, but at least not as if through a glass darkly. Such a week went well with the blooming of the daffodils and with the scent of the crab-apple blossoms that wafted along our street in Silver Spring.

With the comings and goings of my debilitation, I began to see my life imaged in the Greek myth of Persephone, the girl carried off by Pluto to Hades. After a major custody battle between Pluto and the girl's mother, Persephone was condemned to spend half the year underground. Her mother, Demeter, the goddess of the harvest, shows her grief at the absence of her daughter by bringing the deadness of winter. When Persephone returns, spring comes. Periods underground in the kingdom of the dead alternate with green and fertile intervals when the warm light caresses the land.

There is nothing like returning from the dead, I thought, as I strolled among the early-blooming tulips, to make one grateful for life. I imagined Persephone thinking the earth such a wondrous, brave new world that others, never confined to the darkness, regarded her excitement as strange. Likewise, there is no time of year that seems more miraculous than spring, so full of flowering, and coming as it does after the dead of winter.

"Do we always get aware of things through privation?" asks Bernard Berenson in his journal. The aging man has discovered how formidable can be distance, something which had "scarcely existed" for the younger Berenson when he traveled on foot. Only now, when he is easily fatigued, does he recognize what a blessing it was to possess the vitality he previously had.

Another response is possible, and it is often reported by those whom illness or time has humbled. Seeing how delicate is the thread that ties us to life, some come to have a heightened gratitude for whatever of life's blessings still remain. "One of God's mercies" is what Flannery O'Connor called the interval of sickness before death, the time of being diminished but not yet disappeared. "It is through the mercy of survival," she says, "that we learn to admire the birds of flight, the copper tree, the winter light."[26] Grateful to the cosmos for the privilege, however brief, of seeing its wonders, of being a part of its shimmering dance.

Another shift in our relationship to the cosmos can occur: from holding on to control to going willingly with the flow. In the terms of imperialism, the empire-builder can learn the art of surrender. The fear she had of losing control in life, reports Lois Jaffe as she deals with her terminal leukemia, is at the heart of her fear of death. Facing death, she reports that "being in control is no longer of overriding importance to me." Giving up the need for control has led her to a paradoxical discovery: the more she gives up her insistence on being in charge of her life, the more autonomous she feels.[27] Perhaps the empire-building gets in the way of coming into possession of one's being.

In their study *Vital Involvement in Old Age,* Erik Erikson and his collaborators draw upon a Hindu image to represent a positive adjustment to aging. It is the image Hindu philosophy uses "to describe the final letting go—that of merely being. The mother cat picks up in her mouth the kitten, which completely collapses every tension and hangs limp and infinitely trusting in the maternal benevolence."[28]

What are the benefits of such trust? A passage from the Taoist sage Chuang-tzu provides a suggestion: "A drunken man who falls out of a cart, though he may suffer, does not die. His bones are the same as other people's, but he meets his accident in a different way. His spirit is in a condition of security." Under the impact of events that demonstrate the limits of our mastery, we may be led to see the wisdom of such spiritual teachings.

"If such security is to be got from wine, how much more is it to be got from Tao [the way]," says Chuang-tzu.[29] And says Erikson: "The kitten responds instinctively. We human beings require at least a whole lifetime of practice to do this."[30]

But it is not just "practice" that teaches, for practice is usually the repetition of our habitual means of coping. What teaches is the disruption of those habits, the impact of experiences—whether chosen (as in the deliberate pursuit of spiritual knowledge) or un-chosen (as in enduring the impact of illness or aging)—that bring us into collision with the limited adaptive value of those habits.

In this way, it can be those very bumps along the path of life that injure us that can also bring us closer to the Tao.

As I grew smaller—under the impact of a deep, ongoing experi-ence of finitude—my perspective seemed to change.

A few months after our move to the mountains, we went to our first real community event in the area. It was a private affair to which most everyone who lived along this ridge or in the nearby little valleys seemed to have been invited, as well as a number from the hosts' church. Some of the people were from nearby towns and villages; others were farmers. The dress was casual, from jeans and cowboy boots to khaki slacks and red blazers. The hosts' place was their weekend retreat, though unlike most weekenders they lived in the Shenandoah Valley. A red rail fence of wood surrounded the yard, a half-mile down the ridge from our place. Just inside the fence was a smoking pit in which a whole pig had been cooking since the night before. It was a congenial gathering centered around eating barbecued pork from the pig, although every family there had brought a "covered dish" to contribute to the feast. Officially it was called the Pig Roast, though in my usual fashion I dubbed it the Pig Out.

I liked being with the people, even while being profoundly aware that I was in the midst of a very different tribe from my own. How would I fit on their maps, with me descended from Eastern European Jewish ancestry, bred of urban people and intellectuals, while my new neighbors had grown out of rural German Lutheran roots?

I don't usually think this way, unlike people in my extended family of an earlier generation, closer to the Old World outlook. But the recent news about concentration camps in Bosnia had heightened my awareness of tribal differences among neighbors and lent to it an especially paranoid flavor. Women were being raped and men being murdered by people who were their neighbors in little villages. These atrocities were not all committed by strangers against strangers. In Bosnia, people who grew up together, families that intermarried, were turning against one another on tribal lines. In my mind, witnessing this marriage of familiarity and ferocity raised the most disturbing questions. How can peoples living together ever feel secure that their common humanity has overcome ancient fears and hatreds? If burying tribal animosities for two generations' time does not put out the fires, what would be time enough? At the Pig Out, I wondered as I looked into the kindly faces of the four or five generations gathered there together: Are these people's hearts any different from those of the Serbs whose crimes are daily being seared into our memory?

But then something interesting happened. I continued to see the people through the paranoid prism of the nightmare that is currently coming to the world's surface. But I felt close to them anyway. In this, I saw the footprints of my confrontation with illness and mortality. Something had shifted that smudged out what might have once seemed clear lines of division. Even if terrible crimes do lurk as a potentiality among us, I felt that we were all caught up in something that transcends who does what to whom. I saw everyone there, regardless of tribe, caught up in the transcendent cycle of dust to dust. It was like that old Renaissance idea about how, in the grave, there is no difference between the king and the pauper.

In their work about the stages of life, John Kotre and Elizabeth Hall cite the work by Arnheim on the changing perspective of artists in their later years. Older artists, Arnheim found,

> develop a detached contemplation that changes their approach to their craft. In their work, they transcend outward appearances and search out underlying essentials. The result is a world view in which similarities outweigh differences and in which the power of a common destiny pervades the figures on the canvas—even the torturer and the victim in Titian's "The Crowning with Thorns," for example.[31]

Half a lifetime ago, cleavages meant more to my heart. I recall the evening that my brother, Ed, did the Tarot cards with me, and the uncanny way a single card kept coming up: the Knight of Swords, a hard-charging young man on a warhorse, dashing forward with his glinty steel blade ready to slash. This was at a time I was ready to take on the world, and, though I tend to disbelieve in magical synchronicity, that Knight of Swords card did fit well my spirit of that time. For some years I identified with that figure wielding the means to divide good from evil, right from wrong, the problem from the solution, our side from their side.

I have no quarrel with that young man. But I am he no longer. I have learned too much about wounds to take delight in swords.

CHAPTER 7

Welcome to the Human Race

How Illness Can Deepen the Human Connection

The guy next to me still had a bit of the barn on his boots. Chickens, I thought I could discern. The "Oliver North" button on his hunting jacket spoke further about how different his world was from mine. His face had that impassive Clint Eastwood quality—the face, I thought, of a guy who is a stranger to his feelings.

The kindergartners on the stage started their song, and I directed my attention back that way. Nathaniel, who could carry a couple of pieces of firewood a lot better than he could carry a tune, was putting his heart into it. That's my boy! I thought, my own heart filling with what in Yiddish is called *nachus*. If I designed Christmas cards for Hallmark, I noted to myself, I'd put that face on one. A moment later I glanced over at the farmer with the chickens, and the sight of his face stopped me. Looking stageward where, presumably, one of the cherubs was his, the man was beaming. If the stage had not already been lighted, his blue eyes and wide smile would have illuminated it.

He's a father, just like me, I told myself—once again struck by the obvious. Fifty years from now, both of us will be dust. But here we are together beaming pride at the fruit of our loins, channeling them our love to help carry them into a future beyond our own years.

The song ended, and we all began applauding. "Great kids, huh? Which one's yours?" I asked the guy with the North button.

TWO WORLDS REVISITED

For any of us, illness and dying present both challenges and opportunities concerning how we connect with, or separate ourselves from, our fellow human beings.

One possible outcome of our confrontation with our finitude is that we can transcend our division. But this does not happen by itself; it represents a spiritual achievement. Powerful psychological forces are operating in the other direction. Under the impact of suffering and disablement and the fear of death, one may also separate oneself. The wounded and weakened spirit may turn in on itself, forfeiting its sense of connection with the wider human flow.

Just as an injured animal slinks off into the solitude of the woods to nurse its wounds, the ill person may turn inward. As the body under frigid conditions allows the extremities to grow numb in order to maintain the vitality of the body's core, so under the stringencies of debilitation will the psychic energies of the stricken person detach from the outside world to muster the necessary strength to overcome the burden of illness.

A consequence of this can be a kind of narcissistic self-involvement. "How sickness enlarges the dimensions of a man's self to himself!" wrote the famous eighteenth- and nineteenth-century English man of letters Charles Lamb. "He is his own exclusive object." Having as his only duty the "supreme selfishness of thinking 'but how to get well,' " Lamb writes, the convalescent is unaffected by what happens beyond himself.[1]

While on the one hand, the inward turning of one's energies may be an adaptive response to the challenge of recovery, at the same time this "supreme selfishness" appears also as a kind of spiritual disability to compound the enfeeblement brought about by the somatic illness. Lamb presents the case of the sufferer who, before becoming ill, had been greatly concerned about a lawsuit that threatened a friend with financial catastrophe. But now he lies abed, "as indifferent to the decision, as if it were a question to be tried at Pekin." From overheard whispers, he gathers that the suit has been decided, and his friend is now ruined: "But the word 'friend,' and the word 'ruin,' disturb him no more than so much jargon."[2]

The loss of vital powers is often experienced as a kind of narcissistic injury. Until one faces up to the spiritual challenge of coming to terms with the diminution that illness and suffering can bring— not only the loss of vitality, but the heightened awareness of vulnerability as a mere "speck of dust"—this narcissistic wound can sap one's capacity to love and to care for others.

For Betty Rollin, receiving the diagnosis of breast cancer and undergoing a mastectomy were wounding experiences. At the psychic level, as well as the physical level, healing had to occur before she could resume normal living as a member of her human community. Rollin tells of a call she received from a friend, some time after the mastectomy. They discussed some personal difficulties the friend was contending with, involving her boyfriend, her kids, and other such things. "We hung up and, as I started cooking dinner, I tried to figure out what she should do about everything and what, if anything, I could do to help. . . . It occurred to me that I was doing something I hadn't done for a long time. I was worrying about someone else."[3]

By bitterness also can the ill, the disabled, and the dying separate themselves from others. Aldous Huxley depicts a scene in which he visits the hospital room of his cancer-stricken aunt Mary.

> Or rather with the person who had once been Aunt Mary, but was now this hardly recognizable somebody else—somebody who had never so much as heard of the charity and courage which had been the very essence of Aunt Mary's being; somebody who was filled with an indiscriminate hatred for all who came near her, loathing them, whoever they might be, simply because they didn't have cancer, because they weren't in pain, had not been sentenced to die before their time.[4]

When I began researching for this book, I knew I would want to learn more about Beethoven and how he dealt with his deafness. My wife's best friend, Diane Merchant, is herself hearing impaired and teaches music at Gallaudet College, the well-known institution of higher education for the deaf in Washington, D.C. Diane told me that she knew someone there who had herself studied Beethoven's life, and Diane offered to get from that other person at Gallaudet some bibliographic suggestions for my research. When many weeks went by and no such suggestions arrived, I asked Diane what was happening. She had encountered a problem, she told me: when the other person learned that the person who would be using her counsel was a hearing person, she was reluctant to provide assistance.

The hostile division between an "Us" and a "Them" can come from either direction.

Then there is the isolation brought about by shame. The "stigma of illness" opens up a chasm from the operation of two forces. On the one side is the ostracism to which the ill are subjected by the healthy: the healthy want the leper out of sight. But the ill can also share the stigmatizing judgment, feeling too ashamed of their condition to dwell among their fellows.

"How would it be possible for me to admit of a weakness?" asked Beethoven out of shame for his deafness. His solution to his dilemma is self-imposed isolation: "I am obliged to live like an outcast."[5]

Our society's powerful emphasis on self-reliance can also drive the ill or dying to isolate themselves. In that autobiographical literature on illness, the dread of dependency is a recurrent motif. This dread is connected with shame. In the Eriksonian model of development "the tension between autonomy and shame/doubt" is a fundamental issue in the human life cycle. But while shame over the loss of autonomy—incurred, for example, through "bodily damage from illness or injury" or from "the deteriorations of old age"[6]—may be a general human problem, the burden of such shame is doubtless of greater intensity in a culture like ours that especially values the ruggedness of the individual who stands on his own two feet.

A good case of this is Herbert Howe in his triumphalist memoir about his battle with cancer. In *Do Not Go Gentle,* Howe recounts what happened after his initial treatment with chemotherapy. The chemotherapist asked him:

> "Is someone picking you up?" It was a statement more than a question.
> I buttoned up my sleeve and slowly stood up.
> "No. I'm taking the shuttle bus back to Harvard."
> "Why didn't you ask a friend to come and get you?"
> It was a difficult question to answer—self-reliance not to bother friends. . . .
> "I thought I wouldn't need them."
> She drew in her breath and shook her head. "I wish

you the best of luck. But next time, you dumb turkey, arrange to have somebody pick you up. I think you're going to start learning what friends can do."[7]

Howe goes on to describe his nightmare of a trip home. (It is not clear to me whether Howe ever concurred with the assessment of himself as a "dumb turkey" for his determination to lean on no one, that he ever truly learned what friends can do, or whether he remained attached to his pride in self-reliance. The heart of his account is the story of how he defied medical counsel—eschewing the recommended therapy and driving himself relentlessly in a program of exhausting physical exercise—and fared better against his cancer than most patients with his prognosis.) John Wayne binds his own wounds and, if necessary, ties himself to his horse to keep from falling off.

How we experience the universal burdens of illness and death is greatly influenced by the cultural field in which we live. When it comes to our connection with the web of humanity, many of us internalize an ethic of hypertrophic autonomy—better to stumble painfully home on one's own than to ask for help—and all of us must operate in a society where many powerful forces work to fragment the human community.

Why does the community in modern industrial democracies "feel less and less involved in the death of one of its members"? This is a question Philip Ariès asks in his *The Hour of Our Death*. Ariès gives as one reason that the community "no longer has a sufficient sense of solidarity; it has actually abandoned responsibility for the organization of collective life. The 'community' in the traditional sense of the word no longer exists. It has been replaced by an enormous mass of atomized individuals."[8]

To grow ill, and to die, in such a society can be particularly frightening. At the same time, and by the same token, it is also in such a society that the confrontation with our finitude can be a particularly significant opportunity to transcend the atomism our society teaches as human reality. It is a time when we can reexamine how much of an island any one of us truly is or should wish to be.

THE NEED FOR CONNECTION

I have a friend who sometimes stays in touch and sometimes doesn't. I have learned, after years of our friendship, that if I don't hear from him he is probably especially in need of a friend. It is more than twenty years since the last time he was married and now, in late middle age, he laments having no children. He is also an extremely accomplished public performer, a professional who pushes himself hard and, as they say in sports, plays with pain. When things are tough for him, he stops making contact. After our phone conversation—which I will have initiated—he will often say something about how good it was to talk to me. I'll ask, "Why don't *you* call *me* when you're feeling down? You always do feel better afterward." He'll respond: "That's not the way it works."

In *Facing Death,* Robert Kavanaugh prints an extended and moving account written by a woman dying of cancer. This woman describes how big an obstacle in the way of her coping with her illness was her fear of dependency. "Dying also frightened me because I would become a burden to others," she writes. "I was an independent cuss, the doer in our house, the giver on our block. I never learned the art of receiving graciously." She had learned what our culture teaches about the value of independence and about the costs for one's status of being in the receiving role. Illness required her to adopt a posture in the world contrary to those teachings: "I forced myself to ask for things and learned to swallow my shame." But then she found herself able to transform the old definitions of giving and receiving, to use the calamity that had befallen her as an opportunity to grow closer to people. "I cannot tell you how thrilling it was to learn new ways to express my love."[9]

She does not indicate that she came to revel in her dependency; rather, what she accentuates is her discovery of new ways to preserve her old role as the one who gives. "I never dreamed how much the helpless could offer others from a sickbed." Her relationship with a neighbor girl of eighteen illustrates how she combined her new, unsought role as the dependent one with the old role as the person who helps others. "We grew to love and need each other in a wonderful way. I watched this bashful girl blossom in her new sense of purpose, and instead of feeling beholden, I learned to revel in my new role as benefactor, knowing my burden had helped cultivate her new beauty."[10]

Stewart Alsop, a Connecticut Yankee, also had a strong independent streak. "Ordinarily, I rather like being alone," he writes. Cancer compelled Alsop to learn how strong is our need for one another when fear and weakness undermine the foundations of our independence. With a "killing cancer," Alsop says, "you become terribly dependent on other people, and the physical presence of other people becomes essential to you." He learned this from the "awful loneliness" he felt when his wife left his hospital room briefly during his first stay. "[O]n the rare occasions when I was alone those first ten days at NIH I hated it."[11]

Many philosophers have declared that each person is, inevitably and fundamentally, alone. Although asserted as a general existential fact, this notion seems to be particularly applied to the times of our suffering and our dying. No one can ever really feel the pain of another. Each of us must, in reality, die alone.

In her account of her attendance upon her mother's dying, Simone de Beauvoir writes: "The misfortune is that although everyone must come to this, each experiences the adventure in solitude. We never left Maman during those last days which she confused with convalescence and yet we were profoundly separate from her."[12]

But I don't think this contains such great wisdom, and de Beauvoir's own statement supplies a clue to the limits of her case. So the daughter was separate from the dying Maman. Perhaps it is because the experience was, at an important level, profoundly unshared: while the daughter knows the mother is dying, the mother is—presumably deliberately—confusing her dying with convalescence. Two people with two very different realities can be separate even while in the same room.

Such separation can result from denial by the patient or, as in an example described by Orville Kelly, denial by the family. Kelly was brought in to deal with a dying man who would not talk with members of his family. In Kelly's conversation with the patient, the man complained that they "made him feel guilty" for his acceptance of what was happening to him. His wife, he said, would exclaim, "Please! Don't talk like that! You're going to be home with us for Christmas!" As a result of their attitude, "he refused to talk with them any longer."[13] Thus did he dramatize the separation that their different realities had created.

To say that sharing life's painful times is difficult for people to manage is not, however, to say that it is impossible. There may be obstacles to overcome—in accepting facts, in allowing feelings—but if they are overcome, the "adventure" need not be experienced wholly in "solitude."

In the case of the dying man with the denying family, for example, Kelly goes on to relate a happy ending—happy not in providing a victory over death but rather in reopening the human connection.

> When I explained why he refused . . . the sister
> went into her brother's room. . . . When she exited

from the room she was crying, but she told me they had finally been able to hold each other and they cried together for the first time.

"I'm so glad I'm finally able to be honest with him—and with myself," she told me.[14]

Perhaps there is an irreducible sense in which "We each die alone" is true. But there are degrees of aloneness, and the degrees certainly matter—both for the dying and for the bereaved. That study about the acceptance of death which was cited earlier as showing that the intensity of physical pain is a major impediment to acceptance also found that the human connection is a major facilitator of a positive adjustment. Those dying people are most likely to come to terms with their condition who experience "a feeling of great interest and concern on the part of one's nearest of kin and local clergyman."[15]

Connection matters. Indeed, for us human beings—creatures whose sociality is our most fundamental adaptation, whose distinguishing intelligence is itself probably derived from our species' investment in communicating with each other—it may well be what matters most.

When our son Nathaniel was an infant, he was what is called in some circles a "high need baby." In his first six months, he was frequently uncomfortable for reasons not always fathomable by his parents, and his distress could best be relieved by physical contact with one of us, and especially by nursing. On one occasion, when Natty was experiencing distress in a more or less public situation, a woman ventured, on hearing him cry, "He must be hungry." Then, when nursing settled him down, she declared, "Yes, that was it," though his mother, April, knew that at that moment little in the way of material nourishment was being exchanged. The exchange was really of a very different kind of sustenance.

I recalled this scene recently while reading about the care for the dying in the hospice. The hospice movement places a different emphasis from our conventional hospitals in its understanding of what the dying need. Consider the provision of fluids and nutrition. "Drips and tubes may seem a quicker and more efficient way to keep up a fluid intake," writes Herman Feifel in his description of the hospice approach, "but at this stage personal contact matters more than electrolytes and can give refreshment where, before, everything was drought and isolation." In the hospice, the "scientific" medical technique is subordinated to a more human approach. Thus, in the hospice, "many people, families included, are seen to be giving food and drink, slowly and kindly." What is important for these dying people, as for little Natty at the other end of the life cycle, is not so much the material stuff being taken in as the human bond through which the exchange is being made. Thus the hospice works to see that the fluid and nourishment are "given in a manner which draws them near to others."[16]

Just knowing that someone is there with you can make an important difference. For Stephen Rosenfeld's dying father, the son found, "just sitting there, listening attentively, shifting in the chair very little if at all, letting my father proceed at his own pace, countenancing long periods of silence—that this created an almost palpable calm."[17] It may be that nobody else can walk that valley for us, but it is not true that we need to walk it entirely by ourselves.

Whenever life inflicts its heaviest blows upon us, the fibers of human interconnection can fortify us. Without them, we are like the concrete without the steel reinforcements that keep it from buckling.

A study of ninety men and women who had suffered the loss of one or both parents between the ages of two and seventeen found that such loss made these people, as adults, more than usually vulnerable to depression. But not all of them were equally vulnerable. The single factor that most differentiated the more from the less depression-prone, the study showed, was "the kind of care and support the child received from other family members in the wake of loss." Specifically, "the more emotional support and understanding the child received at the time, the less likely he or she was to fall prey to depression later in life."[18]

Even pain is changed, is made more bearable, by the human connection. Arthur Kleinman tells an affecting story about a seven-year-old girl he helped treat during his medical training. Terrible burns over most of her body made this girl's daily life in the hospital a torment. For Kleinman, too, it was excruciating simply to witness the girl's agony. "I could barely tolerate the daily horror: her screams, dead tissue floating in the blood-stained water, the peeling flesh, the oozing wounds, the battles over cleaning and bandaging." Then, one day, came a turning point in Kleinman's approach to the girl: "I made contact. At wit's end, angered at my own ignorance and impotence, uncertain what to do besides clutching the small hand, and in despair over her unrelenting anguish, I found myself asking her to tell me how she tolerated it, what the feeling was like." This empathetic reaching out surprised the girl, who then started to tell him of the experience. "While she spoke, she grasped my hand harder and neither screamed nor fought off the surgeon or the nurse." Each day, Kleinman and the girl would continue this intimate sharing of suffering. The girl, Kleinman thinks, became "noticeably better able to tolerate" her treatments. As for the young doctor, Kleinman reports he learned the therapeutic value of that kind of sharing of the patient's experience.[19]

Norman Cousins has noted a paradox regarding medical training in our country. Different domains of training are regarded as either "hard" or "soft," Cousins writes. The "hard" label, which he terms a "benediction," is applied to subjects like biochemistry and anatomy; whereas subjects like patient-physician relationships "tend to labor under the far less auspicious label 'soft.' " The irony is that "a decade or two after graduation, there tends to be an inversion. That which was supposed to be hard turns out to be soft, and vice versa." By this, Cousins means that the "hard" knowledge base is "constantly changing," while the soft intangibles "turn out to be of enduring value."[20]

Surely, the increasingly sophisticated medical technology for dealing with the human machine is of great utility in treating the ills that afflict us. But the needs of suffering humanity are not all to be treated at that sophisticated level of technological interventions based on scientific understanding of biologically understood mechanisms. Our ancestors have suffered for millions of years, and from those eons have grown into a nature that can draw healing strength from that most ancient of medicines—the loving support of one another.

The mending of the fabric of the human community requires, therefore, that the worlds of the healthy and the sick be bridged and melded into one. The ill person is challenged not to close off from the contact; the healthy, to remain fully present to the suffering other.

BUT FOR THE GRACE OF GOD

As illness generates in the ill person an especial need for the human connection, so also can the experience of such suffering foster in the one who has suffered an enhanced capacity for compassionate contact with other people.

A kind of spiritual progression can issue from the processing of one's own suffering. In the acute phase, illness can drive the circling of one's narcissistic wagons. As in Lamb's case, the words "friend" and "ruin" can lose their meaning in the murky sea of self-involvement. But, after the initial crisis has stripped away one's customary sociality, out of grappling with one's own suffering one may become open to a deeper, perhaps more universal connection.

There but for the grace of God go I. Once one has been pared down to one's barest essentials—a creature of flesh and blood, vulnerable to suffering and yearning for joy—one's kinship with one's fellow creatures becomes more palpable. It becomes clearer that we are all in the same boat, all just different versions of the same thing. One's narcissistic caring for one's separate self can grow into a more comprehensive compassion for all of suffering humanity.

I stopped at the stand of the old farmer over on Route 717 and in addition to the pumpkin and eggs I bought, and the overripe tomatoes the old farmer let me glean from his fields for free, I got a glimpse of another change—a welcome change—that seemed to be happening in me.

The old farmer, I saw, was walking with difficulty. "Hip," he told me in answer to my sympathetic question. "Got it replaced ten years ago and now the damned thing is falling apart." He told me of his frustration at not being able to pick his crops from a reasonable posture. "What really bugs me is when I pitch over onto my face." But he's too old to have the hips replaced again, he said, and so he is stuck with the hips he's got, and the pain that goes with them. I felt his unhappy resignation, his sense that his life as he has lived it for over seven decades is coming to a close.

At the level of the words exchanged, I wasn't sure it was so different from a conversation I might have had in the past. But at the heart level, it seemed I was more deeply there *with* him in his pain. And there was something in the way his eyes met mine that led me to think that he felt that my heart was with him, and that it made a difference.

This change in me I sensed was part of the fruit of my coming to terms with my own illness and the suffering it had brought me.

Clarence Hamilton's anthology *Buddhism: A Religion of Infinite Compassion* recounts the famous story of the transformative experience that set the pampered prince Gotama on the path toward his Buddhahood. Having been sheltered in the palace all his years, the young Lord Gotama at last ventures out and comes in turn upon a decrepit old man ("afflicted and long past his prime"), an ill man ("fallen and weltering in his own water"), and finally the funeral pyre for another man ("neither mother, nor father, nor other kinsfolk will now see him, nor will he see them"). It is his discovery of these inevitable afflictions of human life that instigates the spiritual search that eventually gives rise to that religion of "infinite compassion." In each case, the young Gotama is able to make the connection with his own destiny: "Am I too subject to old age," "Am I too . . . subject to fall ill," "am I too then subject to death."[21]

In her statement in Berman's collection *The Courage to Grow Old,* Anne Marx describes the transformative experience she had with her cancer and her trips to the radiologist's waiting room several times a week. "Here I began to care about the other patients, men and women of every age, race, and circumstance. We talked to each other like sisters and brothers." As a result of this regular encounter with this fraternity of fellow sufferers, she found "a total, all-encompassing compassion." Now that her treatments are finished, Marx reports, she remains changed: "I feel an overwhelming identity with a mighty force of commiseration and kindness, never experienced to such a degree before."[22]

In such ways can the blows that diminish us also make us larger.

Depending on how we process the experience of illness, we may become—like Huxley's Aunt Mary—channels of spiritual sickness or we may become agents of healing. It is this latter possibility that gives rise to the notion of "the wounded healer."

The young boy born with a defective heart and eventually made whole by heart surgery is eager to give back to others who must contend with what he has had to face. "When I get older I'd like to go to hospitals and talk to kids who are getting ready for heart surgery. I'd like to put confidence in them," he says. "I'd like to tell them how glad I am to be alive and about all the great things I can do now that I'm healthy."[23]

This boy has something to give, not least because he has it in him to want to give it. His illness has given him a healer's heart. Regrettably, modern medicine—with its version of our civilization's alienating cult of objectivity—knows not the value of such a heart: "Throughout our training we learn *not* to empathize with the sick," writes Siegel. Despite the failures of the training, as Siegel also observes, "the best doctors are often those who have been seriously ill themselves."[24] Best, probably, because their experience has been transmuted into a compassionate identification with the sufferings of others.

A portrait of a great doctor is presented by Kleinman. As a boy, Paul Samuels developed asthma, a chronic problem that has plagued him since. Now a doctor, Samuels believes that his experience with asthma has made him "a more compassionate and effective caregiver for the chronically ill." "He is not infallible or someone from another planet," says one of Samuel's medical colleagues. But, that same colleague maintains, "he is a model of what is best in medicine." What makes him special is his "humanness," which this other doctor believes has been deepened by his own chronic illness. "He knows what it's like to be there himself." A patient expresses his appreciation: "Dr. Samuels cares what is happening to ya. . . .

Ya feel good just bein' with him. . . . The symptoms, the pain it gets less listenin' and tellin' him."[25]

One does not need to be a "health professional" to contribute to healing. The caring, the listening and telling, the really being there that make Dr. Samuels special in his profession are available to every person in our day-to-day dealings with each other. The opportunity to become more human is always there.

Out of the Small Self

I have a friend who is my friend despite his politics. This fellow came from socially very modest origins, and by sheer dint of will—combined with natural ability—has made himself a highly accomplished professional. He is continually butting his way through obstacles, continually providing proof that he has made something of himself. I admire his achievement. Our conversations about politics prompt me to think about his self-making will, for he seems so completely identified with his own mighty will that his reflexive response to social and political issues is to demand of all in our society that they solve their own problems, as he has, and to object to any obstacles being placed in the way of the expansion of our technological dominance of the planet.

Watching the spiritual shift that has been taking place in me, under the impact of my illness, I have begun to realize that I have been more like my friend than I have always been able or willing to perceive.

I always derived some satisfaction from people telling me how much they admire my taking on the problems of the world, how they could never endure continually facing such painful topics as war and environmental destruction. At the same time, I've often thought the admiration misplaced. I couldn't do what a lot of them do. I have been struck with awe to witness a nurse who can remain, day after day, cheerful and patient and caring while she gives various decaying people sponge baths, spoon-feeds the toothless, changes bedpans.

My energy, characteristically, has been drawn to the plight of the victims of injustice. Those suffering from the vicissitudes of "nature" generally did not engage my guts. I wished the afflicted well, but there has always been a part of me, I think, that felt, "I'd rather be dead than live like that myself." My illness has helped me see that I, like the warriors who prize their honor more than their lives, have identified with my own more powerful part, rejecting and pushing down that part of myself that would remain even if illness stripped me of my powers. All my life, the Nazis have represented for me the depths of human evil—but I could discern a part of me that could comprehend the impulse to eradicate "defectives."

Now that was changing. I started to see that a person is a person, that at bottom it is as simple as that. When Natty was conceived, we did genetic testing (April was on the thirty-five-year-old borderline), but maybe we needn't have. What would have been so intolerable about having a Down's syndrome child, anyway? The powerful self of mine that I had always chosen to identify with is but a smaller self, a narcissistic construct. By diminishing that powerful part of me, I thought, perhaps this illness has enlarged my vision of who I am, who we all are.

I was still no Mother Teresa, but from where I was now standing I could see a bit better than I used to just where she's coming from.

In the waiting room of the radiologist, Anne Marx comes to care about people across the spectra of age and race and class, becoming "much more concerned with all of suffering mankind." Most of us tend to make judgments about what makes a person "worthwhile."

Often, it is "people like us" who are seen as having a value lacking in others. Or perhaps people of greater ability or accomplishment. Or people who "earn" our regard by living their lives according to standards of decency.

In Steven Petrow's book on the AIDS epidemic, there is an account from a woman, involved with much of the seamy side of urban life in America, who rallies to the aid of a former boyfriend who had abused her. He is dying, most horribly, of AIDS, and she tries to use the newspapers to find a place where the man could get the care he needs.

> The only replies we got were threatening phone calls: "He's a nigger, let him die" or "He's a junkie, let him die," as if this was a crime in itself. I mean, the man's a man. If I can forgive him for whatever he did to me, who are you to judge him? Who are any of us to judge him?[26]

Kleinman gives us another story from his own learning process as a doctor. The story concerns a man who, as an adult, had suffered permanent brain damage, and who was under Kleinman's care on an outpatient basis. Each week, the man would come to Kleinman's clinic to report on how things were going. Each week, he would say essentially the same thing. Though, as it turned out, these weekly visits were the high point of the man's week, from Kleinman's point of view they felt like a relatively unproductive use of time. One day, a snowstorm delayed Dr. Kleinman's arrival at the clinic, so that by the time he got to work, the usual amount of work needed to be accomplished in less than the usual amount of time. Under this time pressure, Kleinman told the patient, who had been waiting for several hours, that his appointment would have to be abbreviated. The man, named Paul Sensabaugh, "looked so terribly hurt, like a disappointed child." What hurt him, says Kleinman, "was my brusque manner and the shortening of his allotted time." Kleinman did not want him to feel so wounded, so he tried to explain his own dilemma. "That's OK, Dr. Kleinman," the man assured him.

> I'm accustomed to it. I'm just a small person. I'm hardly a grownup anymore. I know the truth. [Now the sheepish grin had left his face and he was crying.] I'm not all together up here. I'm a half-wit like they said, aren't I? . . . Maybe I should live in a home, you know what I mean, a home for people like me.

Dr. Kleinman reports his reaction:

> I felt a deep sadness break like a wave. I think my eyes teared; I may well have cried with him. Then I felt anger—not at Paul, fortunately, but at the injustice experienced by the weak, the timid, the vulnerable in a world of maneaters. . . . I couldn't help feeling that it was me, not Paul Sensabaugh, who should have felt shame.[27]

These are the last words of his chapter "The Stigma and Shame of Illness."

I was having another one of those "insights" that might represent either wisdom or folly—I couldn't tell which.

I found myself able to connect in my heart more readily across generational—as well as other—lines. People much older, or much younger, than myself no longer seemed so "other." This strengthening of the bridge applied particularly to older generations; I was once younger myself, and so I had previously found it easier to connect with younger people. I found myself thinking, as though it were some kind of profundity: "A person's age is simply a function of when he or she happened to be born." This idea, though a mere tautology on its face, I experienced as a variant of "There but for the grace of God . . ."

This profundity brought to mind another I used to have back in the days when I was buddies with Jason the cat. He and I were very close, though of course we never had the kind of conversations I generally value in my friendships. Sometimes I would be struck by how different he was from me: not only did he not use language at all, he also walked on four legs, ate by putting his face directly into the dish, as well as other anomalies. But my feeling of kinship and closeness to this furry fellow was deeper in my heart than my apprehension of these differences, and sometimes I would affirm this closeness by pronouncing to myself the profound observation: "Jason simply happened to be born with the body of a cat."

FOR ALL BEINGS

When people feel "a sense of attachment to the human flow, to both their biology and their history," write Robert J. Lifton and Eric Olson, there comes with it "a *sense of immortality* which enables active, vital life to go on" despite the knowledge of individual mortality. This sense of immortality, Lifton and Olson say, does not involve "denying the reality of death" but rather derives from a feeling of connection, or participation, with "ongoing life."[28]

For those confined to the small self of the self-isolating individual, the finitude of the human life can seem like unmitigated defeat. But for those who connect with the wider currents of life, death loses some of its sting.

"Now I can let go, now I can die," says an old, terminally ill woman on the rooftop of the hospital in Switzerland. The time is spring of 1945, and the patients have been carried up to the roof to hear the simultaneous ringing of bells across Zurich, celebrating the coming of peace at the end of the nightmare of World War II. "I wanted so badly," the woman says, "to live long enough to see peace on earth come back."[29] For a social atom, *après moi* who cares what comes? But for this woman, the fact that humanity is coming back on course allows her to relinquish with a sense of contentment her own personal rivulet in the broad current of human life.

As the ability to identify with those ongoing currents makes the forfeiture of one's own life easier, so also can the confrontation with one's mortality induce an expansion of one's boundaries to include more transcendent identities. Stewart Alsop observed himself finding "new meaning" in his family heirlooms after his own collision with inoperable cancer. "I suppose I took a new interest in my ancestors when I learned that I was statistically likely soon to become an ancestor myself." One has a choice: one path is that of bitterness or defeat from knowing that the "I" of one's individuality will not endure forever; another path is to apprehend and identify with that which endures, that which is passed along from generation to generation.

One young man, a physician, dying of cancer, says that he has accepted "the idea that the death of an individual is really no more nor less than a punctuation mark in the endlessly fascinating conversation amongst all living things."[30] All living things. The wider flow that endures is not confined merely to the human realm. It is not only creatures "like us" that are worthwhile. Even those who are mute have feelings, and deserve compassion. Even those who put their faces right into their food, lacking the fingers to carry it to their mouths, have dignity and value. Even one who walks with four paws on the bare ground can be one's brother.

Alsop had been a lifelong hunter. But as he found himself face-to-face with Thanatos (Death), "I had no desire at all to kill anything." He found God's words to Noah recurring in his mind: "Neither will I again smite any more every thing living, as I have done." His old love of dove shooting became particularly hard to sustain: Because of the way they fly, "very often you know you have hit a dove, which means it will almost surely die, but you don't pick it up." On a dove shoot after his bout with cancer had begun, he eventually found himself missing, "half on purpose." The boundaries of compassion had expanded, and the suffering of anyone is as if it were done unto one's own. "That Saturday night I had bad dreams—there was one terrible dream in which I shot at little Andrew [his young son], and he flopped about on the ground like a hit dove."[31]

That dove, too, is a child of God who just happened to be born into the body of a bird.

One of the texts of Buddhism, from Santideva, expresses the heart of universal compassion:

> O *that I might become for all beings*
> *the soother of pain!*
> O *that I might be for all them that ail*
> *the remedy, the physician, the nurse,*
> *until the disappearance of illness!*[32]

BROADCAST YOUR BREAD UPON THE WATERS

Sometimes, even things that seem endless come to an end.

During the course of working on this book, my malady has largely abated. I never got a diagnosis; I still don't really know what hit me. But for whatever reason, I feel that I am about 80 percent back from the dark and difficult place to which I had fallen. I wouldn't say that my recovery "just happened": various measures I have taken seem to have helped. I've worked on my digestive sys-

tem and eating patterns, done body work, adjusted my neurotrans-
mitters, corrected my sleep cycle: it all seems to have helped. But
my recovery has some of the element of mystery that characterized
my decline. But hey! I'll take it however I can get it.

So, to a considerable extent, Schmookler is back, but it's not the
same Schmookler. Illness changed my spirit, and, while I don't
repudiate what is gone, I happily embrace the new place to which
my long-unwelcome experience has brought me. I feel grateful to
be ready to do some heavy lifting again in my calling, and I observe
that a shift has occurred in the nature of that calling.

Nowhere is that clearer than in the work I do these days on
radio. Two factors precipitated my turning toward radio work.
First, April went on a powerful AM station in our area to be interviewed as part of the promotion of her just-published book *Eating
for Two* on ways for us to eat that are good for the earth. The book
is very gentle and practical, like its author, but on this call-in show
she walked into an ambush of hostile calls from locals who are
rabidly anti-environmentalist. April's a very capable spokesperson,
but she is not readily poised for combat, and it seemed to both of us
that she hadn't really known how to deal with these attacking
callers. At that time, my book *Fool's Gold* had also come out, so I
decided—as a onetime Knight of Swords, and to protect the family
honor—that I'd get onto the show, too, only I'd be loaded for bear
if bear is what I came upon.

At this time also, Rush Limbaugh was rising to the apogee of his
stardom, like some Godzilla of a balloon floating along in the
Macy's parade. I found Limbaugh's impact on our national conversation deeply disturbing, finding offensive far less the substance of
his positions on the issues than the manner in which he presented
them and dealt with those who disagreed with him. It seemed to
me that it is dangerous to bring glib certainties to bear on the
questions we face as a people. There had been talk in America

about the need for something on the left to balance Limbaugh, but it seemed to me that the opposite of "The Rush Limbaugh Show" was not to have the same thing from a different side of the battle lines, but to have a completely different kind of conversation—one not about beating one's interlocutors over the head but rather about working together in a process of genuine inquiry. As if we really might learn something from one another.

One change in me in the wake of my malady was that I felt quite sincerely open to such a conversation. To what extent it was being humbled by my illness that made me feel humbler about the adequacy of my own understanding, I don't know; there is also just getting older and becoming more impressed with one's ignorance than with one's knowledge; and certainly the "liberal" or "progressive" viewpoint had in general wandered into some sort of cul de sac. The likes of Limbaugh treat their adversaries with contempt and scorn, a dynamic that only further tears the social fabric. But besides the adverse consequences, my heart had changed in a way that made it more painful for our public discourse to be conducted in that tone than it would have been before. It now seemed to me that we human beings are all struggling to be good human beings, and to understand the situation we're in, and all deserving of empathy and respect for that effort. Differences in viewpoint, differences in intelligence and education, differences even in our moral uprightness—while they are not unimportant, they seem to me rather secondary to the ways in which we are all—like the torturer and the victim on Titian's canvas—on the same plane.

For these reasons, as I came back to life my greatest desire was to reach out to my fellow human beings in a spirit of caring and questioning to open a dialogue about the issues that we wrestle with in our lives. And when I went onto the "Mid-Day Show" with Jim Britt—on WSVA, 55 on your dial—to plump *Fool's Gold* and to defend the family honor, in the back of my mind was the hope that this appearance might give me the opportunity to begin such a dialogue.

The station sits atop a hill overlooking Harrisonburg, Virginia, and a wide swath of the Shenandoah Valley where a hundred and thirty years before, Yankees had come south to slash and burn the granary of the Confederacy. I settled into the small studio, where the host, Jim Britt, also functions as engineer and answers the un-screened phone calls from listeners. The interview went well. When the ambushers called, I felt able to parry their thrust without having to draw blood. Britt and I talked during the various com-mercials. We're doing good radio, he said. By the time the two-hour show was over, we had agreed that I would come back as a regular guest to talk about "the issues of the day." And I have continued to do so, introduced by Britt as "author and NPR com-mentator," and at my behest now also "talk radio philosopher" and, when I can coax him into doing so, occasionally as "the gadfly of the Shenandoah Valley."

I'm on twice a month, two hours at a stretch. For each show, I prepare a commentary to frame the question for our discussion. The show that felt most pivotal for me in deepening the conversa-tion was the one I was most afraid of doing. I called the show "God Said It," because in it I expressed my reservations about the attitude expressed by the bumper sticker that reads, "God said it. I believe it. And that settles it." After a year of doing the show, that subject just pushed itself upon me, as so often the callers from this Bible Belt region would, if not say precisely that, at least convey that attitude. For me it was a real conversation stopper. And I just could no longer deal with that attitude without finally biting the bullet and confronting it. It was frightening, however, to contemplate what I might unleash on myself.

A huge epistemological gap, as I saw it, separated me from those callers. How do you *know* that's what God thinks? It's in the Bible.

How do you know the Bible is God's word? It says so. What about the Koran, the Upanishads, and other such texts that people in other parts of the world think record what God said to *their* ancestors? Those religions are false. You were born into a Christian household, how would someone from Mars be able to tell which of these texts was truly the word of God and which religions were false? Is there any chance that what God has to say is bigger than any single tradition has grasped, and that we could all learn from each other?

Did we, on that morning, learn from each other? I think at some level, we did. The conversation was a wonderful experience for me and, I gather, for a number of other people. I don't think anyone's mind was "changed" in the usual sense of shifting beliefs, but it was a kind and caring exchange of thoughts: people remained stuck in their belief systems, as far as the words spoken demonstrated, but we also came to appreciate a bit more the struggles of others. On my side, at any event, I felt moved to recognize that—although many of the fundamentalists who called me violated the rules of epistemology and logic that I was brought up to regard as inviolable—the belief system many of these people hold so tenaciously is valuable and important, a core of value and orientation that many who practice my way of thinking sorely lack. The whole issue has caused me to reexamine where, in my overall hierarchy of values, I put the kind of "truth" that people like me arrive at through the kind of thinking that I regard as intellectually responsible. For my listeners, all I can report is that many of them have told me that they appreciated the chance to be part of a conversation like that.

Jim Britt gives me a pretty free hand in choosing topics, and I choose questions that I am wrestling with myself and that I think will be meaningful to the thirty or forty thousand people who are listening. Sometimes it is a political issue, sometimes a moral or cultural issue, or just a personal one. Topics have included: "Brother's Keeper" (when and in what ways should we involve ourselves uninvited in other people's affairs in an effort to help them?); "Racism"; "What does it mean to love one's country?"; "Do people want what is good for them?"; "What experiences have shaped your relationship with right and wrong?"; "Why are people in America so angry with their government?"; and "What should be the role of work in our lives?"

Here are a few moments from the programs that I savor in remembering. One Memorial Day, in the midst of a show on patriotism, a Vietnam veteran, who carries the scars of that war, and I, who protested it in the streets, figuratively embraced each other with respect on the radio. In a discussion of the origin of evil, a pubescent home-schooled fundamentalist boy and I discussed the riddle of why God, who can foresee everything, would have created an Adam he would have known would disobey the commandment not to eat of the tree of the knowledge of good and evil. When we were discussing how we should—and how we shouldn't—protect our children from the dangerous and toxic aspects of our world, a mother and I discussed her way of dealing with her eight-year-old daughter's asking, "What is abortion?"

I go into the carpet store to place an order for a strip of Astroturf, and the salesman takes my credit card. "I should have recognized the voice," he says, looking at my name. "I tried calling your show this morning but couldn't get through." It was that program about when we shouldn't just mind our own business. "I wanted to tell you about how I handled a situation at McDonald's this weekend. Some young guys were using foul language—loud. There were families with kids in the place. I dressed those guys down pretty good, but it didn't help. It almost came to throwing punches. I wanted to ask you if you thought there'd have been a better way." So for the next ten minutes, we talk it over. As I leave, he points to the Astroturf and says, "Don't worry, Andy, I'll make sure they cut it right."

I live now in the Shenandoah Valley. A Yankee in the heart of the Confederacy. A Democrat in a region that votes to the right even in the Republican primaries. A Harvard-educated globalist intellectual in a provincial region of farmers and shopkeepers. A grandson of Russian Jews among the Christian fundamentalists. A son of the Enlightenment in the Bible Belt. And never in my adult life have I felt that I had so meaningful a connection, and role, with the community in which I live.

PART III

Finitude

CHAPTER 8

The Final Act

What Is the Meaning of Death in Our Lives?

So, I'm mortal; I'll not be here forever. Same with you. That's not news, I guess, since it was always so. What is news for me is the extent that—at least some of the time—I recognize in my guts that it is true.

What difference does this knowledge make? Will this knowledge act, as some say, as a "worm at the core" of my life? Will knowing that death will come cast a shadow over my days? Or can that knowledge in some way enhance my life?

Clearly, whatever the potential value of being mindful of one's death, it cannot be classified as good news. Otherwise, I wouldn't have done so well the first forty-plus years of my life at keeping that knowledge at bay.

CONTEMPORARY RESISTANCE

Death has always been problematic for human beings. But our present civilization seems to resist the idea of mortality with especial fierceness.

One reason that is proposed to explain the particular difficulty that people in modern society have in coming to terms with death is that we are less familiar with death than our ancestors. Not only have the dying been removed from the home to more isolating institutions, but changes in life expectancy have rendered death more of a stranger. "In our time," writes Johann Hofmeier, citing a study by Alois Hahn regarding death statistics in Germany and Sweden, "a person must be fifty before he experiences the same number of deaths [in the family] as a twenty-year-old in 1820."[1] This idea makes some sense: I recall that the death of my father, when I was twenty-one, occasioned the one big boost in my understanding the reality of our mortality before my own chronic illness. The less one is forced to confront the brutal facts of human finitude, the more one is able to entertain the illusion of one's immortality.

The fact that "direct contact with death and dying has become rarer"[2] has limited explanatory power, however. It may be true that the average person in our society is seldom exposed to the dying, but this is not true of the people in the medical professions. Yet, although these professionals are continuously confronted with the reality of human mortality, they do not appear to be free of the general resistance. Josef Mayer-Scheu interprets as "an unconscious expression of their defensive attitude to death," the behavior of a group of nurses observed in a study of how they responded to different groups of patients. What was observed was that the nurses hurried when called by patients whose condition was improving, but delayed responding to the calls from those "on the threshold of death." When a patient accepts his coming death, Ariès says, this acceptance is apt to be rejected by those who tend him. Most modern medical practitioners, according to Ariès, have repudiated the image of death as "a phenomenon of nature," turning it instead into a kind of alien and accidental force that must be "brought under control."[3]

If it were simply a lack of contact with death that impairs our acceptance of the naturalness of death as a part of human life, one would expect those who see it every day to have different attitudes from the rest of us, whose lives are more sheltered. But, as Philip Kapleau observes in his work on the Buddhist view of death, the medical profession (despite its continuous confrontation with mortality) reflects the general "cultural pattern" in its determination to "thwart the death process." Although, according to Kapleau, death "ought to be welcomed as natural and inevitable," like the rest of society, doctors look upon death as "the great enemy . . . the terror of all terrors."[4]

In Kapleau's description of this cultural pattern, there may lie a clue about the modern rejection of death. Along with the fierce determination to conquer death, Kapleau sees a tendency to regard "all pain as pointless." Perhaps something in how we in modern society tend to regard life, and its purposes and meanings, helps explain our difficulty in accepting death. If life is regarded in hedonistic terms, as seems increasingly the case in our affluent, consumerist society, what meaning can death have? Earlier I discussed the notion that illness and suffering have no place in the American Dream. Perhaps the way we construe life likewise has difficulty accommodating the fact of our finitude.

Another possible factor is that our difficulty is an outgrowth of a change in the way we construe what happens when we die. When I think of death, I see it as simply an end, the termination of being. Creatures come and creatures go, bubbling up from the sea of life. A bubble bursts, and although the substances that compose it endure—the stuff that made the watery film and the gas that it encapsulated are still part of the universe—there is no more bubble.

This image of death as final and complete governs much of the feeling I have about my own dying.

I recall at my high school graduation being surprised that they called it a "Commencement": I thought we were celebrating being finished. But I could see how finishing high school also meant beginning the rest of our lives. I'd feel rather differently about dying if I could see my graduation out of life as a kind of commencement.

But I cannot. How can one believe in the immortality of the soul after one has seen someone disappear into the darkness of Alzheimer's? In such a case, the soul didn't even seem to survive as long as the body, let alone continue after the body's dissolution. What I think of as my "soul"—and what I would think worthwhile to have survived my death—has seemed an inconstant presence even in my own life.

The "death of my soul"—or at least its lapsing into somnolence—for days at a time was the hardest part of this illness to accept. During those years, of course, it showed an ability to be reborn when the cloud lifts. But this rebirth seemed attributable to the resilience of the organism, like being able to walk again after an injury heals. I would not expect to be able to walk again once my legs are dead and buried in the ground, returning to the earth. Likewise, if all my chemistry were decomposing, what kind of soul could I have? If the soul seems to disappear when one is prostrate with salmonella, how is it going to survive death?

Throughout this work, when I have considered death I have assumed its absolute finality. No life after death. This seems by far the simplest and most plausible way of viewing human life; the notion of an afterlife is cut away by Occam's razor. This is an assumption, however, that I continue to question. How, after all, can I be certain? Is there any weighty evidence on the other side?

What about that feeling that we are more than our bodies? It appears through history, across cultures. I have that feeling. Does this represent some intuitive insight into a reality we do not otherwise apprehend clearly? Perhaps. But I am inclined to interpret it as a manifestation of a disconnection within ourselves, of a failure to integrate our consciousness with the body of which it is the fruit. It has been suggested[5] that our neocortex is not well-connected with our more primitive (but absolutely vital) brain structures. Perhaps this contributes to a sense of a detachable consciousness. Even if the tendency toward disconnection is not anatomically based, we have been swept along in a historical process that creates a war between societal injunctions that we learn to internalize and natural inclinations that are embedded in our flesh. The result is a tendency to identify with the acceptable part, which has entered into us from the surrounding world through our consciousness, and to reject what is forbidden (inherent in the natural body). To me, it is no wonder if people have historically entertained the illusion that their real selves were somehow separable from all corporeal being.

Some people are persuaded by the evidence of near-death experiences, or apparitions of the dead, or out-of-body experiences. Perhaps if I had experienced any of these, my beliefs about death would be influenced by them, also. But I have not, and I have no idea whether to regard these phenomena as illusory or as a clue to there being more in heaven and earth than is dreamt of in our naturalistic philosophy.

One line of thinking, however, does give me greater pause. If only fools believed in a notion that seemed to me highly implausible, it would be easy for me to dismiss it. But with life after death, it seems quite otherwise. It seems to me precisely those who, on other matters involving the human spirit, seem the most wise who, generally speaking, are most often proponents of the idea of life after death. In some cases it is a survival of the soul in a different realm, as in Western religions, while in others it is an Eastern cycle of death and rebirth. But whichever, I cannot but be impressed when an idea that seems to me incredible is advocated by many of the leading religious teachers of human history, people who, on other matters on which I feel in a better position to judge, seem to have a deep and illuminated wisdom.

This gives me pause, but then I go on believing that death is annihilation.

COLD COMFORT

If you believe in an afterlife, is death easier to take? In my materialistic view, dying means losing everything. Even with the best of scenarios of an afterlife, admittedly, dying would require saying good-bye to a great deal. Like graduation from high school, even going on to higher things does not wholly eliminate the sadness of taking leave of old friends and leaving behind an important phase of one's life. Nonetheless, I would expect that, on the whole, death is easier to accept if it is seen as a transition to a new existence than if it is regarded as a cessation of existence itself.

As we will see shortly, the belief in an afterlife can have some disturbing aspects, but the proposition that it is on balance a comforting belief is supported by a study that found that this belief is most prevalent among the dying. While only a third of a control group in this study believed in the possibility of an afterlife, fully 84 percent of a group of dying persons did so. There is no need to be afraid of death, says the Buddhist Roshi Yasutani: "we are indifferent to death, since we know we will be reborn."[6] For the survivors, too, belief in a hereafter is comforting. "I have the need to believe that my son exists somewhere," says one bereaved mother. "My belief is based on my emotional need and not on my reasoning."[7]

The belief in an afterlife came considerably easier in earlier eras, when religious orthodoxy predominated and when the scientific perspective on human and other life was less developed. If more people in our times understand death as mere annihilation, instead of as a threshold to a new life, perhaps this change in belief helps account for any increased resistance among modern people to the idea of mortality.

Nothingness is hard to take. It is hard enough for a lot of us to be reconciled to the idea that "you can't take it with you." The idea that you aren't going anywhere, even without it, is even harder to bear.

FINAL EXAM

On the other hand, belief in an afterlife can bring burdens of its own, making the time of dying frightening in different ways. For some, the idea of an afterlife includes the possibility of eternal damnation. Some tormented imaginations have foreseen eternal nightmares that make oblivion look like paradise by contrast. But even without the nightmare of hell, belief can add to the stress of dying: death can be transformed into the crucial moment, the culmination of the whole life.

"The salvation of man is determined at his death," was the old Christian belief.[8] "In that instant the dying man has the power to win or lose everything," as Ariès sums up this high-pressure perspective. Kapleau articulates a parallel idea from the Buddhist system of belief: "Your state of mind at the time you draw your last breath is crucial, for upon this hinges your following rebirth."[9]

Death becomes a kind of final examination. All one's prior work can here bear fruit—or come to naught. Like most final exams, this kind of death could be filled with anxiety.

Brother Damien is dying painfully of multiple sclerosis. As Buchanan tells in *Patient Encounters,* Brother Damien, his life having been spent in a monastery in the pursuit of the purification and salvation of his soul, feels "haunted, taunted and toyed with" by his pain. His main fear, Buchanan tells us, is that "his illness would undo in a single moment of agony all the spiritual work that it had taken him years to accomplish."[10] As if dying in pain were not enough of an ordeal, Brother Damien's belief system makes his dying still harder. As Philippe Ariès states the old Christian view of death, it is "an ordeal that is being given to the dying man, an ordeal whose outcome will determine the meaning of his whole life."[11]

But what if we discard the belief in an afterlife? What if we see death as simply the point at which the temporary aggregation of matter and energy that we are begins to disaggregate? What is the meaning of death, then? What is the meaning of death as an *event* in our lives, after which we are no more? And what is the impact of the knowledge that this is what our lives must come to on our lives preceding death? What does such a death do to our lives and to the question of life's meaning?

WHERE ARE THE DEAD?

When I think about the moment a person passes into oblivion, I find some paradoxes in my own belief.

My wife, April, is reading a novel. (When April is reading a novel, she always keeps me posted. It is one of the fringe benefits I enjoy for having replaced her journal when we got together.) In this novel, *Damage,* by Josephine Hart, the protagonist is having an affair with his son's fiancée. Toward the end of the novel, the unsuspecting son inadvertently discovers the two together. Recoiling in horror, the son stumbles backward over the railing of a stairway, and falls to his death.

When I hear of this incident, I am filled with anguish imagining how I would feel in the father's position. How terrible it would be if my son's *last moment* was poisoned with the sense that I had betrayed him! It would be bad enough for him *ever* to feel that I had done him wrong, but worse if he were to die with that ill feeling between us. I couldn't stand it.

But then I am impressed with the apparent illogic of my reaction. As events unfolded in the novel, the son's feeling of betrayal lasted only a few seconds. Then it was gone, for the one who bore the feeling existed no more. What does it matter if that was the *last* feeling? How would that greatly alter the entire picture of a relationship that had otherwise been characterized by positive feelings? Would the history be so very different if the son had been struck and killed by a car a half an hour before? It seems that I am imagining the last moments continuing in perpetuity, out of reach of revision. A bad feeling that can never be made right.

Since my two older children were rather young, I have had joint custody of them. My time with them alternated regularly with time we were apart. Each time they were with me, I made a point to attend to our final moments together. It was important, I felt, what feeling was left between us for the days until we were together again. Those feelings would endure in their young hearts—would continue to glow or fester—to flavor the time we were apart, and I wanted to do what I could to make that residual connection feel happy and strong.

That attention to parting moments made sense in that situation, I think. But is it not paradoxical, if one believes dying to be complete annihilation, to give as much importance to parting words as I know I, and most other people, do?

Simone de Beauvoir reports finding a similar paradox in herself. Writing of her going to her mother's deathbed, she says: "I did not particularly want to see Maman again before her death; but I could not bear the idea that she should not see me again. Why attribute such importance to a moment since there would be no memory?"[12]

Even in our rather secular society, we do not regard the deceased as though they were gone as well as dead. In our property law, we honor the wishes of the dead—even at the expense of the living—as if the dead still had a stake in our actions, as if they still had active interests.

If death is annihilation, it would seem to follow that the dead have no real "interests." Among people who believe that the dead are simply gone, therefore, would a "rational" property law disregard the expressed will of the deceased whenever it varies from the interests of the living? Arguably not. For one thing, destructive chaos might ensue in the world of the living if people lost faith that their will would be done with their property after they were no longer present to see to it themselves. But more important, from a psychological standpoint, the dead are meaningfully present in the hearts and minds of the living, and it fills an important emotional need of the living to honor the memory of the dead. If our property law treated those who have died as merely so much water and carbon and nitrogen and calcium, as organic molecules that are in the process of decomposition, the living would feel impoverished.

Is it perhaps in the survivors alone that a death has meaning? If the deceased has returned to his primordial speckhood, does how he died matter at all only because it matters to those who maintain the temporary quintessence in their dust?

Norman Cousins tells the story of getting involved in the dying of a judge. The judge's defeatism in the face of his cancer, seeming so uncharacteristic of whom he had been, threw his whole family into despair. After an effective intervention by Cousins, the judge rallied and, for the sake of his family, was able to die in the larger and more courageous way he had lived, to die "in character." After the judge's attitude shifted, his wife reported to Cousins: "The ultimate outlook hasn't changed, but the general atmosphere has. We are . . . well, a lot less despondent than we were." And Cousins concludes: "He was able to govern the circumstances of his passing in a way that provided spiritual nourishment to the people who loved him. He died in character. This was his gift to everyone who knew him."[13]

Similarly, Grof and Halifax note how reconciliation and closeness and mutual participation of the dying person and the family "in the process of dying can take away much of the despair of the survivors."[14]

Death here is not a final examination to determine the future destiny of the departed, but the "how" of dying matters nonetheless, for the event lives on in the memory of the survivors. Depending on how the leave is taken, the survivors can be left with peace of mind or with unresolvable distress. For a loved one to die feeling betrayed, as in the novel my wife was reading, leaves a burden on the survivor—not to have apologized, not to have reconciled. I have myself witnessed a grief made much more difficult by the death having occurred at a time of conflict in a relationship that had for many years before been quite loving: the survivor is left with a final dissonant note reverberating that cannot be resolved into harmony. That is why I have always counseled friends to make their peace with their aging parents while it is still possible.

This all makes emotional sense: people's feelings do work this way, and so the counsel is good. Yet beneath this psychological sense, do I still detect some logical nonsense? While the living need to make their peace with the dead, is not that need based on some fundamental denial—or a fundamental inability to comprehend—that the dead are not around to make peace with?

At one level, my relationship with my father has continued to evolve in the years since his death. Some of that occurs through dreams. The year after his death, I had one dream that was particularly vivid and even exhilarating. I was a king visiting some other kingdom. As I was about to retire for the night, I came to know that there was a plan afoot to assassinate me. My position's like Duncan's in *Macbeth,* I recall thinking in the dream, but I'm not going to sit here and await the fate they're planning. I stole out of the castle by some secret passageway that, somehow, I knew about. The castle had been dark, but outside it was no longer night. Mediterranean light suffused the scene. In front of the castle there were chariots to rent, and I found one belonging to Phil Silvers. We haggled over the price; he drove a hard bargain as well as a chariot, but I got a price I liked and we took off. The land inclined gently downward toward an azure sea, and we headed downhill, gaining speed. As the wind generated by our rapid progress whipped through my hair, I suddenly knew with exaltation that I was speeding to join my father. To celebrate, I withdrew from my cloak two wind instruments and held them up to the wind and, as the wind blew through them, with my fingers I played the lyrical Allegro movement from Bach's "Musical Offering." My father and I shared a great love of Bach, and it was a fitting piece to celebrate our coming reunion. I woke up from the dream as if relieved of my grief.

But was not the notion of a reunion promised in the dream basically a comforting illusion—the illusion that there is still someone to be reunited with? My dead father still appears occasionally in my dreams, and it is always a big deal to see him. I feel he is still a part of my life—not just my memory of him, but *him.* But that feeling is logically incompatible with my intellectual belief that there is no longer any such being as Jacob Schmookler. Is not our emotional landscape but an internal Gettysburg, filled with monuments to our fallen dead, monuments made of stone and metal made to create the illusion that the dead are made of permanent stuff?

And if we, as survivors, have such difficulty grasping the death of others as complete annihilation, is it not much more difficult to come to grips with the meaning of such a death at the end of our own lives?

COME TO NOTHING

If I am about to cease existence forever, what difference does it make just how I make my exit? One way people find answers to such a question is by aestheticizing their lives, by regarding their lives as if they were works of art, with a form that can be more pleasing or less. Just as the death of a loved one should represent a "happy ending," so might one strive to make of one's final chapter a fitting closing to the life that has gone before. "People with integrity affirm that their story was a good story," wrote Kotre and Hall, "with continuity from beginning to end—and true to the person who was its author."[15]

Life as a work of art. I can appreciate that as a solution to the problem of how to give meaning to one's death, and life. But the idea of the work of art also calls attention to the human propensity to embrace illusion as reality. One can become quite agitated with the hope that Romeo will intercept the friar, bearing Juliet's message, and so avoid their heartbreaking fate. Our agitation bespeaks our ability to forget, at least in part, that the course of events has already been determined. Even more than that, we are able to suspend our knowledge that the two star-crossed lovers are fictitious. They never were.

Do we similarly fool ourselves when we think it matters, after our deaths, whether we ended our story well? But even more disturbing than that is another question. Once we are in our graves, does it matter how good any of our story was? The ancient Greeks had a saying that no man should be called happy until he succeeded in preserving that happiness until his death. But not only is it unclear why happiness at that last moment should matter, in view of our destiny to return to dust, is it clear of what significance it is whether our lives were happy or not along the way?

Living posthumously, as I was for so long, I wrestled with feelings of futility. If I will lose everything in the course of time anyway, what difference does it make what I get or do on my way to the grave? But I couldn't tell whether this was a logical *non sequitur*. It is easy to see how, in that state—living posthumously—the notion of the futility of everything might seem more persuasive than it deserves. When, in terms of how I felt inside, the sight of glowing clouds on the mountaintop moved me no more than the sight of a concrete wall, no wonder "What does it matter?" could seem a question about life in general that may have no good answer. But I did think I knew better than that.

There is, however, something about the finality of death that raises questions about whether life matters. I recall facing some puzzles along these lines, even in brighter days, and I've always had difficulty wrapping my mind around them.

When I was in high school in the early 1960s, Pope John XXIII died. He had seemed to be a wonderful man, and it really distressed me to hear that in his last hours he had been in terrible agony. It hurt to think of so good a man suffering so much. Then the thought occurred to me, now that he's dead, what difference does it make what agony there was a few hours before? It's over, it's not happening now, it's the same as if it never happened. Although that argument seemed somehow flawed, it also seemed somehow irrefutable.

Similarly, when I would read history. A painful episode—like the massacre of a village, or the ripping apart of a family—would cause me distress, and then I would think: that was a hundred years ago; they'd all be dead anyway. What difference does it make that Abraham Lincoln lost his beloved Ann Rutledge? They would in any case both be dust now.

That way of looking at the implications of our finitude in time seemed occasionally to take the edge off the pain of contemplating the tragedies of the past. Its logic, however, would also eviscerate life of its positive meanings. "Nothing matters" would be a pretty dismal and empty conclusion to reach about life.

Does death's inevitability and finality imply life's futility? I'm not the only one to have pondered that logical step.

"One event happeneth to them all," saith the voice in Ecclesiastes, thinking of our ultimate destiny in the grave. "Then I said in my heart: As it happens to the fool, so it will happen even to me. . . . And why was I then more wise?"[16] If time will destroy all one's achievements, if it will sweep away all one has made of oneself, what is the use of striving to do or to be anything at all? The British philosopher F. C. S. Schiller sounds like the Ecclesiast when he declares that "to assert that death is the end of all beings is to renounce the ideal of happiness, to admit that adaptation is impossible, and that the end of effort must be failure."[17]

"You are back where you started," laments the composer Hector Berlioz near the end of his life, contemplating how the cycle of dust to dust renders one's achievements futile.[18] "One returns to nothingness," says a twenty-one-year-old female college student interviewed in a study on attitudes toward death, "and then it is as if one had never existed." Death makes one's efforts "so futile, so worthless, so absurd."[19] And the British philosopher W. Macneile Dixon declares that death makes whatever one does a "wanton waste of energy." If all of us die, "all values, truth, goodness and the rest, go with them into everlasting night, no theological or metaphysical twitterings can rebut the demonstrable hollowness of life, its inherent futility."[20]

The same logic I employed to console myself about the pope's suffering renders history into but so much sound and fury, signifying nothing. Gwynne Dyer contemplates the ancient battle of Megiddo, and then declares: "It is impossible to care much about who won the battle, because both sides lived long ago and far away, and most of what they cared for—their family and friends, their language, their religion, their personal and political hopes and fears—has vanished utterly." Dyer recognizes that this is not the way we regard the events of our own times; these we imagine to be great and full of significance. That, says Dyer, is the way we feel "about the Normandy invasion of 1944, but if history goes on long enough, the day will come when Megiddo and Normandy will seem on a par: equally futile and equally meaningless."[21]

For us mortal beings, according to this argument, death renders all our imputations of meaning mere illusion. Because our lives are finite in time, they are necessarily hollow and futile.

This argument, although at moments it has appeared to me hard-headed and persuasive, is itself hollow and unable to stand up.

THE ONLY ITEM ON THE COUNTER

For a while in my adolescence, I was a compulsive photographer. Unless I took a picture of some life experience, it hardly seemed real to me. I'd climb to the top of a hill overlooking the Mississippi

River a ways south of Winona, Minnesota, to see the stunningly beautiful sweep of the river, and the hills of Wisconsin on the other side. But to see this beauty was somehow not enough. I needed to make something *lasting* out of the event (if not a picture, a poem would suffice); otherwise it just happened and was gone, and was therefore empty. I examined this compulsion, this need or greed to accumulate embodiments of my experience, to see if I could discover what it was about. Ultimately, I saw, the need for the photos grew out of something missing in my relation to my own experience. It was because I was unable to be fully present in the experience itself that I wanted some enduring sign of the experience to stand as an assurance that the experience persisted, *for so long as it persisted I hadn't missed out on it yet.*

The fallacy at the root of the case for futility lies not in the argument's view of death but in a fundamental misorientation toward life. There is a kind of greed operating here, a greed that insists on holding firm to something that is inherently flowing. This greed leads to the spiritual fallacy that only what is permanent can matter.

The term "greed" seems applicable, for this kind of psychically compensatory mechanism underlies also the insatiable materialism of our civilization. George Santayana called money "coagulated happiness," meaning it is an external manifestation of an internal experience that has not occurred. About this I wrote in *Fool's Gold,* in the section called "Indian Giver":

> We live in the richest country in the history of the world,
> but it seems we're always hungry for more—as if our
> things were themselves so much stored-up happiness. As
> if money, embodying all the gratification we have de-

layed, or been incapacitated from experiencing, were a promissory note that promised a future of fulfillment.[22]

But happiness must be experienced within. And so, too, must the meaning of our lives. Experience, like music, occurs through time. For those disabled from fully dancing to the music of their lives, time will inevitably be seen as the bearer of futility and failure. Only permanence would seem to offer a solution.

But this solution is really no solution, even if it were possible. Just as the billionaire's stockpile of "coagulated happiness" does not bring happiness, but only perhaps the means of evading the confrontation with one's disability, so would everlasting life not solve the problem of futility that some attribute to the fact of our mortality.

Consider a mathematical way of looking at it. If it were true that our lives amount to naught because they are finite, what would that imply about the meaningfulness of an eternal life? If a human life span is empty, would that not imply the same if our lives lasted a thousand years, or a billion? If $70 \times x = 0$, where x is the meaningfulness of each year of our lives, then 1 billion $x = 0$. For evidently, $x = 0$. And if our lives never ended, just when would our lives become meaningful? If it happened some place along the way—say at y years—then meaningfulness is achieved also if we were to live $y + 1$ years. And if meaningfulness never happens at any finite time, but only at eternity, then it never happens at all, for we never reach infinity. (This leaves aside the fact that infinity times zero is zero.)

If our three score and ten are futile, then so would lives lived immortally. It makes no sense to say that death makes life futile, for all death does is to remove future possibilities. If the present has no meaning, then neither would an indefinite future; if the present does have meaning, it is of the same kind as if our future went on forever.

I recall reading a historical account of the beginning of the Cold

War. Someone criticized President Truman's policies, saying that he was "only buying time." I do not recall who wrote the passage, but I do recall his defense of Truman, for it seemed to me to reflect real wisdom. Time, he said, was the only item on the counter.

Time flows, and so our experience of it is inevitably of finite increments. Even if it never ended for us, this would be so. In the struggle between meaning and futility, fullness and emptiness, therefore, death is not the issue. The heart of the matter is, rather, how we live our lives.

NOW

What is finite is finite. The image of Aristotle's ephemera, cited earlier in the quote from Montaigne to suggest how brief is a human life, can cut the other way. What does it matter how brief—seventy years or a billion? Time is time, and the now is all there is. ("Is a lily for a day worthless? Should sunsets be canceled because even the most glorious don't last forever?" asks the aptly named Gardiner Moment.)[23] Now, the precious moment.

How does one face death? Consider the famous Zen story of the man, pursued by the tiger above, harassed by the dragon below, holding onto a cliffside by a root that his weight is extracting from the ground. Spotting a ripe strawberry near his hand on a ledge, he plucks it and savors its flavor: "How delicious!" he exclaims. Recall that woman, dying of cancer, who enjoyed, though she could not swallow, her food. Her last words before going to bed the night she died in her sleep she spoke after marveling at the colors as the sun sank beneath the horizon: "What a magnificent sunset!"[24]

It doesn't matter if we have x days to live or y, says Bal Mount facing terminal cancer. "We're all in the same boat." Each day, says Mount, we're all one day closer to dying. "For all of us then, it isn't the quantity of life but the quality that counts."[25] Orville Kelly recounts the day he broke out of his funereal way of relating to his terminal diagnosis. He realized, "I was alive! . . . I had some time. . . . What is a day, a month, a year. . . . [O]ne more day would be a lifetime."[26]

Siegel says that medical personnel sometimes look askance when they hear laughter booming out of the room where Siegel is conversing with a dying patient. They suspect, says Siegel, that Siegel and the patient are "denying reality." But Siegel invites them to the realization "that people aren't 'living' or 'dying.' They are either alive or dead."[27]

LOVE AND FAREWELL

Who has the harder time facing death? Those whose lives have been rich and satisfying? Or those who have had difficulty also in facing life?

The Stoics evidently thought that the less we lose, the easier it must be to give it up. To dissuade others from their fear of death, they used the argument that life is no great thing. Christian writers, too, "have insisted on such a devaluation of life as a remedy for the fear of death."[28] Conversely, in his discussion of attitudes toward dying in the later Middle Ages, Philippe Ariès argues that the main difficulty people of that era had in dealing with death was that they were so in love with life, so zestful in their pursuits, that they could not stand the thought of surrendering it all in death.

It seems sensible that this is how it would be, that those who love life would cling desperately to it and those whose lives are unfulfilling would be more inclined to welcome, or at least to accept, the coming of death. But the workings of the human spirit are not always so straightforward. The opposite may be the more powerful relationship.

Said Confucius: "One who sees the Way in the morning can gladly die in the evening."[29]

"The idea of death made my head spin because I didn't love life," writes Sartre about his childhood. And his longtime lover, Simone de Beauvoir, observed similarly: "The evidence I have shows that the fear of death does not generally coincide with an ardent love of life: on the contrary."[30]

Just as death will appear to render life futile to him or her who has not lived it fully, so will the person who holds back from life be mortified by the prospect of death. The great psychoanalyst Otto Rank, discussing the fear of death in the neurotic, connects it with a fear of life. The way he puts it is that the neurotic refuses "the loan of life in order to escape the payment of this debt (death)."[31] But this formulation, I believe, puts it backward, making the fear of life a strategy to cope with the fear of death. I expect it is rather that the fear of death is the by-product of the incapacity to live in a fulfilling way. "I think my own fears of dying are really disguises for my fears of living," says Lois Jaffe.[32]

In his book *The Wheel of Death,* Philip Kapleau presents another Zen story that recalls the strawberry on the side of the cliff. A roshi is dying and, being given a piece of his favorite cake bought for him at a Tokyo pastry shop, he begins to munch on it.

> As the roshi grew weaker, his disciples leaned close and inquired whether he had any final words for them.
> "Yes," the roshi replied.
> The disciples leaned forward eagerly. "Please tell us."
> "My, but this cake is delicious!" And with that he died.[33]

EATING ONE'S FILL

We all have to leave the table sometime, but most bitter is having to leave without having really been nourished.

My favorite time at a restaurant is when I am launching into the appetizer. My appetite is still at its maximum, and I am also eating. (So much for drive theory, which foolishly postulates that our goal is mere drive reduction, satiation.) At the end of the meal, satisfied, I am willing to leave. Those who are just beginning their meals I regard with some slight wistful envy, but I am content. I've had my turn, and those who came later get their turn after mine. I accept being finished.

This restaurant image has often struck me as an apt metaphor for my feelings about the way time carries me through the human life cycle. I was amused, therefore, to find—in two different places in my reading—reports of dreams using a similar metaphor. In one, an elderly woman, nearing death, dreamt that it was time for her to leave the restaurant to make room for others. In her dream, she reported, she felt some regret for having to leave, but satisfied too that her meal had been good. In the other, Lois Jaffe (the woman with leukemia) was hosting a party, and as her guests were about to leave, she realized she had more food she had forgotten to serve. Despite her entreaties that they stay, the guests said they'd had enough and they departed. Jaffe awoke with a feeling of sadness, which she then sought to interpret. What she was sad about, she concluded, was not that she had been a bad hostess, but because "I was so busy entertaining and giving the party that I had not had time to enjoy my own party." This dream led her to change her way of living the time she had left.

RIPENESS

Is there such a thing as *enough*? This is a question I raised in my work on the materialism of our civilization in relation to our cult of economic growth and our apparently insatiable appetite for wealth. But the question can arise also with respect to our relation to the finite span of our lives.

There is a passage concerning death in Max Weber's essay "Science as a Vocation" that has stayed with me since I read it my freshman year of college. Weber's ruminations here are touching, coming as they are from a man who had himself chosen the vocation of science *(Wissenschaft)*, and written as they were at a time in his life when Weber was dealing with personal depression and when he was but a couple of years from his own death at the age of fifty-six. The passage deals with the question of the meaning of death in human life.

To make his melancholy point, Weber draws upon the ideas of Tolstoy, whose "broodings," says Weber, led him to the conclusion that for modern civilized man "death has no meaning." This is so because "the individual life of civilized man"—and here, Weber clearly means also the man devoted to science—is placed "into an infinite 'progress' " and therefore should "never come to an end; for there is always a further step ahead of one who stands in the march of progress." In this orientation toward progress without end, the modern person stands in contrast with "some peasant of the past," such as Abraham. Abraham, according to Weber, "because he stood in the organic cycle of life," could die "old and satiated with life." In terms of its meaning, such a life could have "given to him what life had to offer." But he whose life-meanings are defined in terms of linear progress, instead of organic cycle, can only become "tired of life," not filled and satisfied.[34] For those of us whose view of life is shaped by the culture of empire-building, there is no such thing as enough, no acceptable limit, no possible sense of completion.

Weber's analysis purports to reveal the empty fate of the modern person. This exaggerates the power of the argument, however, for history cannot make us so totally its prisoner. But it does illuminate if not our fate then our dilemma. For we are pulled by powerful historical forces that work to alienate us from the organic patterns of nature.

"Because he stood in the organic cycle of life." The way of Abraham is still open to us, for we are by nature the same as he. Like him, we are creatures born of flesh and blood into a cycle of growing and decaying. It is in our nature as animals on this earth to live, to wear out, and to return to the dust from which we came. The structures that have grown out of our history may be antagonistic to that reality, but they have done nothing to alter it. If Abraham can fall to the earth full of ripeness, so can we.

"I'm a satisfied customer," says the old woman contemplating the span of her years. Siegel tells of his grandfather who, "at the age of ninety-one said, 'Get my friends together and get me a bottle of schnapps. I'm going to die tonight.' To humor him, the family complied. That night after the party he went upstairs, lay down, and died."[35]

Not all of us will be allowed to come to such a ripeness; some are plucked off the tree before the full season is complete. Even if death comes from some acute disease, however, the chance for a feeling of completeness remains. A woman dying of cancer ventured on a psychedelic experience, under the auspices of Grof and Halifax, which enabled her to review her life in some depth. "Everything that has been my life is being shown to me. . . . Memories, thousands of memories. . . . It was such a beautiful life; no one would believe what a beautiful life I have had." After her return to normal consciousness, say Grof and Halifax, she felt a continuing contentment. "The experience made it easier for her to face death, since she was able to recognize and appreciate how full and rewarding her life had been."[36]

Our lives, by nature, are finite. But they are not infinitesimal. Into the limited human vessel, life pours a rich if finite brew of experience. If we can be open to that richness, evidently, we can ripen into a capacity to accept our end.

Not Just Despite

Must the knowledge that we will die gnaw like a worm at the core of our lives? The Zen master with his cliffside berry suggests that life can be savored though death is imminent. Despite the awareness of death, we can still appreciate the beauty of the sunset. No, not just *despite* death. The knowledge that life is scarce can heighten our appreciation. With both diamonds and time, the fact of scarcity drives up the value.

"The consciousness of our mortality is a precious gift," asserted Max Frisch.[37] While "death destroys a man," said E. M. Forster, "the idea of death saves him."[38]

A brush with death can cleanse the soul. When Diane Cole returned from her hostage ordeal, where the possibility of sudden and violent death had hung over her as a constant threat, she found that for her "every color, texture, smell, and taste was discovered anew, with a newborn infant's joy."[39] When Zinsser's R.S. knew that he would soon die, it seemed to him "as though all that his heart felt and his senses perceived were taking on a 'deep autumnal tone' and an increased vividness."[40] And similarly, Stewart Alsop reported a "special euphoria" with his temporary return to life with the ebbing of his cancer's first onslaught. Brighter colors, heightened interest, dearer friends—these are the enlivening changes Alsop relates. In the wake of the discovery of mortality, life continues not just undiminished but enlarged.

Siegel said that there is no important cleavage between the living and the dying, for both are still among the living. Perhaps a more important dichotomy is between those of the living who are in touch with how miraculous a blessing it is to be alive and those who are not.

An inveterate bargain hunter, I sometimes used to think of life as that best-of-all-deals: something for nothing. We didn't have to do anything, after all, to get it. But with time I have found a different metaphor more fitting. Life is a passage we get to book without any advance payment; we do, however, have to earn our way as we go. It is not always cheap. Clearly, not everyone finds the journey worth the ordeal. Some have a rougher trip than others; some learn better than others how to draw value and meaning from whatever occurs along the way. Life, while always a miracle, is not always felt to be a blessing.

But so long as the spark of life remains, the opportunity remains that one may discover the blessing that seems latent in the miracle. Even dying and death, so often seen as our great curse, can be the instrument of this discovery. This surprising potentiality is the underlying theme to which Elisabeth Kübler-Ross points with the title she gives the collection she edited: *Death: The Final Stage of Growth.*

In this collection, for example, Murray L. Trelease recalls "a nineteen year old boy dying of leukemia who in two weeks' time grew from a rather irresponsible brat to a loving, understanding counselor who led his family through the shattering experience of his dying."[41] Later, Mwalimu Imara tells about the transformation of an older woman. At the outset of her terminal stay in the hospital's cancer ward, this woman was "demanding, abusive, foulmouthed, and cantankerous." She had lived "a long life of isolation, possessed by her work, but giving herself to no one." Reminiscent of Huxley's Aunt Mary at the start, this woman changed, at least partly as a result of therapeutic visits from Imara. She became "a joy to visit." Says Imara, "We watched as the sixty-eight year old caterpillar became a graceful butterfly. . . . As she accepted her illness, she became more able to accept the human contact that was still available to her." A month before her death, the woman declared, "I have lived more in the past three months than I have during my whole life."[42]

April has driven to Virginia Beach to see her mother. Fifteen months ago, her mother—Dorothea Moore, née Isaksen, a Swede from rural Iowa—had a heart attack. Lying in intensive care one night, she suffered cardiac arrest. Anywhere else and she'd have been gone, but in that unit of the hospital the monitors picked it up right away and within a minute or two she woke up with a doctor pounding on her chest. For several days, her main feeling about the event seemed to be annoyance at the indignity of being awakened so rudely and at the roughness of the treatment that left her ribs feeling bruised. But ever since she survived that hard bounce off the frozen lake that awaits us all, she has really flowered. She seems really delighted to be alive, and is a delight to be with. Gone are the last vestiges of that heaviness of spirit that clung to her for years after her husband, "Mac," died: his final days were in a convalescent home a mile from where he and Dorothea had lived together, his Alzheimer's having progressed too far for her to be able to care for him, but she'd had trouble forgiving herself for not keeping him at home until the end.

Now she is full of girlish laughter, and I can just imagine how she'll take April out to dinner tonight to a restaurant whose major virtue is that it overlooks the ocean whose motion, even though her vision is failing, she still relishes watching. They'll precede the meal with a gin and tonic, and they'll end the evening swapping stories while performing the ritual that constitutes for the Isaksen girls their own particular "strawberry" of life's high points: a mutual foot rub. April used to wait until the time was right for the whole family to go to Virginia Beach for a visit, but since that close call fifteen months ago she feels a need to go there more frequently.

My own mother just dodged the bullet, too. The biopsy results were favorable, and so she just takes her heart medicine—as she has been doing in the dozen years since her own heart attack—and continues her creative work. The recent scare led her the other evening to tell me just where the keys to the safety deposit box are kept, "in case something happens to me," as she puts it. Talking about death is not, generally, her thing, but I know she hears the clock ticking. I've never found it that easy to get Mom out the door when it was time to go someplace, and I'd bet that Death, when the time comes, will find her pretty stubborn, too. She's got a mind of her own, and there's a lot she wants to get done. But she does sometimes confront the subject of there being a time after her, a time that realism suggests to her cannot be terribly distant.

"When I'm gone, Andy, there will be no one left who *knew* my mother." That thought is full of tragedy for her, a sign of one of the least acceptable aspects of the cosmic order. It was that thought that moved her, not long ago, to spend four years writing a very powerful novel based on her mother's life. I know she worried sometimes she would not have time to complete it, and now she is frustrated that she has not yet found anyone to publish it. But I assure her that the manuscript will be a treasure for me and my children and my children's children, that it will be preserved and with it the memory of Anna Mumlin, her mother.

For my mother, the creative process and family are the two great pillars of meaning, and she is ceaselessly finding ways to weave the two together. As long as she has the energy to stir herself, and so long as her back problem does not lay her out, she goes to her painting group twice a week to do her art—pictures of old men at the Wailing Wall, a wise-looking Caribbean woman with a colorful bowl of fruit in her lap, an old Chinese man reading a newspaper in a doorway, and, especially, portraits of the family. So I am sending her the surprisingly good new portrait of Terra from Wal-

Mart and looking forward to the day, some months from now, when Terra, lovingly rendered by my mother's brush, hangs on Mom's wall, perhaps between the portrait she did of me a few years back and the one she painted from the wedding picture of her parents.

So long as there is life, there remains in us the possibility for the growth of the human spirit and the realization of its potential for beauty. In these, if in nothing else, lies our salvation.

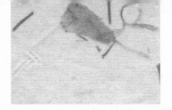

NOTES

Beneath It All There Is No Bottom (pp. 3–39)

1. Betty Rollin, *Last Wish*, p. 8.
2. Norman Cousins, *The Healing Heart*, p. 203.
3. Bernie Siegel, *Love, Medicine & Miracles*, p. 39.
4. Moira Griffin, *Going the Distance*, p. 73.
5. Susan Sontag, in Edwin S. Shneidman, editor, *Death: Current Perspectives*, p. 105.
6. Griffin, *Going the Distance*, p. 93.
7. Paul Levitt and Elissa Guralnick, *You Can Make It Back*, p. 21.
8. Howard Brody, *Stories of Sickness*, p. 112n.
9. Cited in Susan Sontag, in Shneidman, *Death*, p. 104.
10. Bernie Siegel, op. cit., p. 180.
11. Quoted in Sontag, in Shneidman, *Death*, p. 105.
12. Mark and Dan Jury, *Gramp*, p. 55.
13. Arthur Kleinman, *The Illness Narratives*, p. 159.
14. Personal communication with Dr. Anthony Bober.
15. Myra Bluebond-Langner, *Private Worlds of Dying Children*, p. 189.
16. Griffin, *Going the Distance*, pp. 38–39.
17. Barbara Sourkes, *The Deepening Shade*, p. 27, italics in original.
18. Esther Goshen-Gottstein, *Recalled to Life*, p. 14.
19. Harold Kushner, *When Bad Things Happen to Good People*, p. 38.
20. Jill Krementz, *How It Feels to Fight for Your Life*, p. 105.
21. Kushner, *When Bad Things*, p. 15.
22. Ibid., p. 17.
23. Ibid., p. 19.

Living Posthumously (pp. 40–77)

1. Shakespeare, *Julius Caesar*, Act II, Sc. 2, line 30.
2. Philippe Ariès, *The Hour of Our Death*, p. 143.
3. Charles Adler et al., editors, *We Are But Moments*, p. 29.
4. Colin Parkes, cited in Beverly Raphael, *The Anatomy of Bereavement*, p. 290.
5. Betty Rollin, *First, You Cry*, p. 127.
6. Beverly Pitts et al., "Life After Football," p. 3.
7. Arnold Beisser, *Flying Without Wings*, p. 81.
8. Samuel Johnson, in Charles Taylor, editor, *Growing On*, p. 9.
9. *The Sun*, Issue 196, March 1992, p. 9.
10. Moira Griffin, *Going the Distance*, p. 104.
11. See Schmookler, *Out of Weakness*, pp. 136–42.
12. Beethoven, in H. C. Robbins Landon, editor, *Beethoven*, p. 84.
13. Ibid.
14. Janet Maurer and Patricia D. Strasberg, *Building a New Dream*, p. 261.
15. Ousama Ibn Mounkidh, in Taylor, editor, *Growing On*, p. 41.
16. Howard Brody, *Stories of Sickness*, p. 164n.
17. Ibid.
18. In Jill Krementz, *How It Feels to Fight for Your Life*, p. 103.
19. Oliver Sacks, *The Man Who Mistook His Wife for a Hat*, p. 9.
20. Ibid., p. 15.
21. Esther Goshen-Gottstein, *Recalled to Life*, p. 76.
22. Sacks, *The Man Who Mistook*, p. 50.
23. Ibid., pp. 152–53.
24. Paul M. Levitt and Elissa S. Guralnick, *You Can Make It Back*, p. 2.
25. Robert Kavanaugh, *Facing Death*, p. 50.
26. Paul Tournier, *Learn to Grow Old*, p. 180.
27. Beisser, op. cit., p. 81.
28. Stravinsky, in Taylor, editor, *Growing On*, p. 24.
29. Griffin, *Going the Distance*, p. 18.
30. Erik Erikson et al., *Vital Involvement in Old Age*, pp. 194–95.
31. Beethoven, in Landon, editor, *Beethoven*, p. 84.
32. In Landon, editor, *Beethoven*, op. cit., p. 195.
33. Hans Zinsser, *As I Remember Him*, p. 439.
34. Erikson et al., *Vital Involvement*, p. 197.
35. Joseph Heller and Speed Vogel, *No Laughing Matter*, p. 162.
36. Longfellow, in Taylor, editor, *Growing On*, p. 113.
37. Berenson, in Taylor, editor, *Growing On*, p. 32.
38. Myrna Doernberg, *Stolen Mind*, p. 141.
39. Virginia Ironside, introduction to John Rush, *Beating Depression*, p. 9.

40. William Styron, *Darkness Visible*, p. 42.
41. André Gide, in Taylor, editor, *Growing On*, pp. 118–19.

Struck by the Obvious (pp. 78–115)

1. Judith Viorst, *Necessary Losses*, p. 269.
2. Judy Tatelbaum, *The Courage to Grieve*, p. 39.
3. Diane Cole, *After Great Pain*, p. 57.
4. Tony Bober, personal communication.
5. Medlinda Beck, "The New Middle Age," *Newsweek*, December 7, 1992, p. 51.
6. Malcolm Muggeridge, in Phillip L. Berman, editor, *Courage to Grow Old*, p. 255.
7. Harold Bloomfield, quoted in *Newsweek*, December 7, 1992, p. 50.
8. *Newsweek*, December 7, 1992, p. 50.
9. Philippe Ariès, *Western Attitudes*, pp. 86–87.
10. Barney G. Glaser and Anselm L. Strauss, "The Ritual Drama of Mutual Pretense," in Edwin S. Shneidman, editor, *Death*, p. 166.
11. Quoted in Zachary Heller, "Jewish View of Death," in Elisabeth Kübler-Ross, editor, *Death*, p. 46.
12. Zachary Heller, "Jewish View of Death," in Kübler-Ross, editor, *Death*, pp. 46–47.
13. Ron and Jane Nichols, "Funerals: A Time for Grief and Growth," in Kübler-Ross, editor, *Death*, p. 92.
14. Ibid.
15. Ariès, *Hour of Our Death*, p. 580.
16. Robert Kavanaugh, *Facing Death*, p. 16.
17. Geoffrey Gorer, in Shneidman, editor, *Death*, p. 28.
18. Malcolm Muggeridge, in Berman, editor, *Courage to Grow Old*, p. 256.
19. Ariès, *Western Attitudes*, p. 90.
20. Harold S. Kushner, *When Bad Things Happen to Good People*, chapter 1.
21. Charles Taylor, editor, *Growing On*, p. 27.
22. Joseph Heller and Speed Vogel, *No Laughing Matter*, pp. 23, 25, 83.
23. In Lucien Stryk, editor, *World of the Buddha: A Reader*.
24. Stephen Rosenfeld, *Time of Their Dying*, pp. 11–12.
25. Johann Hofmeier, "The Present-Day Experience of Death," in Norbert Greinacher and Alois Muller, editors, *Experience of Dying*, pp. 22–23.
26. Kavanaugh, *Facing Death*, p. 13.
27. Stewart Alsop, *Stay of Execution*, p. 45.

28. Freud, quoted in Robert J. Lifton, "The Sense of Immortality," in Herman Feifel, editor, *New Meanings of Death.*
29. Lucretius, quoted in Arnold Toynbee, "The Relation between Life and Death," in Shneidman, editor, *Death,* p. 11.
30. Ben Hecht, quoted by Robert Kastenbaum, in Feifel, editor, *Meanings of Death,* p. 19.
31. Josef Mayer Scheu, in Greinacher and Muller, editors, *Experience of Dying,* p. 120.
32. Kenneth A. Shapiro, *Dying and Living,* p. 74.
33. C. S. Lewis, quoted in Peter Marris, *Loss and Change,* p. 39.
34. Tatelbaum, *Courage to Grieve,* p. 23.
35. Shneidman, *Deaths of Man,* p. 7.
36. Gordon Stuart, quoted in Arthur Kleinman, *Illness Narratives,* p. 147.
37. Shneidman, *Deaths of Man.*
38. Shneidman, in Shneidman, editor, *Death,* p. 281.
39. Ariès, *Hour of Our Death,* p. 21.

Tethered to a Dying Animal (pp. 116–142)
1. Josef Mayer Scheu, "Compassion and Death," in Norbert Greinacher and Alois Muller, editors, *Experience of Dying,* p. 121.
2. Quoted in Jacques Choron, *Death and Modern Man,* p. 106.
3. Quoted in Judith Viorst, *Necessary Losses,* p. 309.
4. Thomas Bell, quoted by Mwalimu Imara, "Dying as the Last Stage of Growth," in Elisabeth Kübler-Ross, editor, *Death,* p. 149.
5. From the "Anattalakhana Sutra, or Discourse on Not Having Signs of the Self," Clarence H. Hamilton, editor, *Buddhism,* p. 33.
6. Virginia Woolf, *The Moment,* p. 10.
7. Montaigne, in Charles Taylor, editor, *Growing On,* p. 102.
8. Cited in Ernest Becker, *The Denial of Death,* p. 33.
9. Nesson, quoted in Philippe Ariès, *Hour of Our Death,* p. 121.
10. Jonathan Swift, "Cassina and Peter," quoted in Becker, *Denial,* p. 33.
11. Ariès, *Hour of Our Death,* p. 311.
12. Ernest Becker, summarizing idea of Otto Rank, in *Denial,* p. 109.
13. Ira Wallach, in Phillip L. Berman, editor, *Courage to Grow Old,* p. 155.
14. Cited in Leslie A. Marchand, in Berman, editor, *Courage to Grow Old,* p. 287.
15. Ben Hecht, quoted in Robert Kastenbaum, "Death and Development," in Herman Feifel, editor, *New Meanings,* p. 18.
16. *Newsweek,* January 11, 1993, p. 60.
17. Judith Stillian and Hannelore Wass, in Shneidman, editor, *Death,* p. 233.
18. Elliot Jacques, reported by Edmund Sherman, *Meaning in Mid-Life Transitions,* p. 7.

19. James Dickey, in Taylor, editor, *Growing On*, pp. 24–25.
20. Viorst, *Necessary*, p. 270.
21. Cited in John Kotre and Elizabeth Hall, *Seasons of Life*, pp. 301–302.
22. Montaigne, *Essays*, p. 33.
23. Quoted in Viorst, *Necessary*, p. 285.
24. Shakespeare, quoted in Diane Cole, *After Great Pain*, p. 61.
25. Choron, *Death and Modern Man*, p. 214.
26. Robert Kastenbaum, "Death and Development," in Feifel, editor, *Meanings*, p. 28.
27. Ariès, *Western Attitudes*, p. 44.
28. Malcolm Muggeridge, in Berman, editor, *Courage to Grow Old*, p. 257.
29. Ariès, *Hour of Our Death*, p. 130.
30. Montaigne, *Essays*, p. 34.
31. Karyn Feiden, *Hope and Help*, p. 39.
32. Schmookler, *Fool's Gold*, p. 58.
33. Betty Rollin, *First, You Cry*, p. 89.
34. Cole, *After Great Pain*, p. 115.
35. Paul Tournier, *Learn to Grow Old*, p. 171.
36. Thomas Wolfe, quoted in James Buchanan, *Patient Encounters*, p. 76.

Coming to Terms (pp. 143–155)

1. Herman Feifel, editor, *New Meanings*, p. 37.
2. Shakespeare, *Hamlet*, Act V, Sc. II, lines 231–33.
3. Norman Cousins, *Head First*, p. 216.
4. Bernie Siegel, *Love, Medicine & Miracles*, p. 25.
5. Ibid.
6. Raymond G. Carey, "Living Until Death," in Elisabeth Kübler-Ross, editor, *Death*, p. 79.
7. Judy Tatelbaum, *Courage to Grieve*, p. 24.
8. Philippe Ariès, *Hour of Our Death*, p. 579.
9. Stanislav Grof and Joan Halifax, *Human Encounter with Death*, p. 119.
10. Paul Tournier, *Learn to Grow Old*, p. 177.
11. Quoted in Steven Petrow, *Dancing Against the Darkness*, p. 111.
12. Ernest Becker, *Denial of Death*, p. 102.

The Virtues of Our Necessities (pp. 156–175)

1. Howard Brody, *Stories of Sickness*, p. 29.
2. Paul M. Levitt and Elissa S. Guralnick, *You Can Make It Back*, p. 165.
3. Arnold Beisser, *Flying Without Wings*, pp. 132–33.
4. Ibid.

5. Cited by Paul Samuels, who is quoted in Arthur Kleinman, *Illness Narratives,* pp. 211–12.
6. Cited in Suzy Szasz, *Living with It,* p. 57.
7. Robert Lifton and Eric Olson, *Living and Dying,* p. 64.
8. Janet Maurer and Patricia Strasberg, *Building a New Dream,* p. 279.
9. Ibid., p. 275.
10. John McLeish, *The Ulyssean Adult,* p. 235.
11. In H. C. Robbins Landon, *Beethoven,* p. 193.
12. Stanislav Grof and Joan Halifax, *Human Encounter with Death,* p. 107.
13. Robert Kastenbaum, "Death and Development," in Herman Feifel, editor, *New Meanings,* p. 39.
14. Ibid.
15. Karyn Feiden, *Hope and Help for Chronic Fatigue Syndrome,* p. 129.
16. Brody, *Stories of Sickness,* p. 57.
17. Quoted in Lois and Arthur Jaffe, "Terminal Candor," in Feifel, editor, *Meanings,* p. 209.
18. Moira Griffin, *Going the Distance,* p. 119.
19. Grof and Halifax, *Human Encounter with Death,* p. 191.
20. Moira Griffin, *Going the Distance,* p. 91.
21. Robert E. Kavanaugh, *Facing Death,* p. 10.
22. Letter to *The Sun,* Issue 196, March 1992, p. 10.
23. Quoted in "Menopause," *Newsweek,* May 25, 1992, p. 72.
24. Quoted in Kavanaugh, *Facing Death,* p. 51.
25. Quoted in Lois Jaffe, "Letters to Seminar Student in 'Methods of Intervention with Dying,' " in Austin H. Kutscher, Lillian G. Kutscher, et al., editors, *Dialogues,* pp. 28–29.
26. Quoted in Levitt and Guralnick, *You Can Make It Back,* p. 169.
27. Lois Jaffe, "Letters," in Kutscher, Kutscher, et al., editors, *Dialogues,* pp. 36–37.
28. Erik Erikson et al., *Vital Involvement in Old Age,* p. 333.
29. In Philip Kapleau, editor, *Wheel of Death.*
30. Erikson et al., *Vital Involvement.*
31. Quoted in John Kotre and Elizabeth Hall, *Seasons of Life,* p. 378.

Welcome to the Human Race (pp. 176–206)
1. Charles Lamb, quoted in Howard Brody, *Stories,* p. 101.
2. Ibid.
3. Betty Rollin, *First, You Cry,* pp. 156–57.
4. Aldous Huxley, in Charles S. Adler et al., editors, *We Are But Moments of Sunlight,* p. 47.
5. In H. C. Robbins Landon, *Beethoven,* p. 84.
6. Erik Erikson et al., *Vital Involvement in Old Age,* p. 188.
7. Herbert Howe, *Do Not Go Gentle,* p. 65.

8. Philippe Ariès, *Hour of Our Death*, pp. 612–13.
9. Quoted in Robert E. Kavanaugh, *Facing Death*, pp. 48–49.
10. Ibid.
11. Stewart Alsop, *Stay of Execution*, p. 53.
12. De Beauvoir, in Elaine Marks, *Simone de Beauvoir*, p. 111.
13. Orville E. Kelly, *Until Tomorrow Comes*, p. 105.
14. Ibid.
15. Raymond Carey, "Living Until Death," in Elisabeth Kübler-Ross, editor, *Death*, p. 79.
16. Herman Feifel, editor, *New Meanings*, p. 165.
17. Stephen S. Rosenfeld, *The Time of Their Dying*, p. 77.
18. Research by Dr. Alan Breier and researchers at NIMH, cited in Diane Cole, *After Great Pain*, p. 98.
19. Arthur Kleinman, *The Illness Narratives*, pp. xi–xii.
20. Norman Cousins, *Healing Heart*, pp. 141–42.
21. Clarence H. Hamilton, editor, *Buddhism*, pp. 6–9.
22. Anne Marx, in Phillip L. Berman, editor, *Courage to Grow Old*, p. 150.
23. Jill Krementz, *How It Feels to Fight for Your Life*, p. 5.
24. Bernie Siegel, *Love, Medicine & Miracles*, p. 57.
25. Arthur Kleinman, *Illness Narratives*, pp. 211–13.
26. In Steven Petrow, *Dancing Against the Darkness*, p. 66.
27. Kleinman, *Illness Narratives*, pp. 168–69.
28. Robert J. Lifton and Eric Olson, *Living and Dying*, p. 76.
29. Quoted in Elisabeth Kübler-Ross, in Kübler-Ross, editor, *Death*, pp. 122–23.
30. Quoted in Edwin S. Shneidman, in Shneidman, editor, *Death*, p. 215.
31. Stewart Alsop, *Stay of Execution*, p. 211.
32. Santideva, quoted in Clarence H. Hamilton, editor, *Buddhism*, p. xxi.

The Final Act (pp. 207–235)

1. Johann Hofmeier, in Norbert Greinacher and Alois Muller, editors, *Experience of Dying*, p. 14.
2. Ibid.
3. Philippe Ariès, *Hour of Our Death*, p. 587.
4. Philip Kapleau, editor, *Wheel of Death*, p. xvi.
5. Paul MacLean, "The Paranoid Streak in Man," in Arthur Koestler and John Raymond Smythies, editors, *Beyond Reductionism*.
6. Roshi Yasutani, quoted in Kapleau, *Wheel*, p. 8.
7. Edith Mize, in Elisabeth Kübler-Ross, editor, *Death*, p. 101.
8. Quoted in Ariès, *Hour of Our Death*, p. 109.
9. Kapleau, editor, *Wheel of Death*, p. 81.
10. James Buchanan, *Patient Encounters*, pp. 124–25.
11. Ariès, *Hour of Our Death*, p. 109.

12. De Beauvoir, in Elaine Marks, *Simone de Beauvoir*, p. 108.
13. Norman Cousins, *Head First*, p. 25.
14. Stanislav Grof and Joan Halifax, *Human Encounter with Death*, p. 69.
15. John Kotre and Elizabeth Hall, *Seasons of Life*, p. 377.
16. Ecclesiastes 2:13–15.
17. F. C. S. Schiller, quoted in Jacques Choron, *Death and Modern Man*, p. 162.
18. Hector Berlioz, in Charles Taylor, editor, *Growing On*, p. 40.
19. Quoted in Edwin S. Shneidman, "College Students," in Herman Feifel, editor, *New Meanings*, pp. 73–74.
20. W. Macneile Dixon, quoted in Choron, *Death*, p. 172.
21. Gwynne Dyer, quoted in Ira Wallach, in Phillip L. Berman, editor, *Courage to Grow Old*, p. 156.
22. Schmookler, *Fool's Gold*, pp. 57–58.
23. Gardiner Moment, in Berman, editor, *Courage to Grow Old*, p. 227.
24. Quoted in Grof and Halifax, *Human Encounter with Death*, p. 107.
25. Bal Mount, in Kübler-Ross, editor, *Death*, pp. 130–31.
26. Orville Kelly, quoted in Feifel, editor, *New Meanings*, p. 187.
27. Bernie Siegel, *Love, Medicine & Miracles*, p. 44.
28. Jacques Choron, *Death and Modern Man*, p. 119.
29. Confucius, quoted in Kapleau, editor, *Wheel of Death*, p. 76.
30. Quoted in Marks, *Simone de Beauvoir*, p. 125.
31. Otto Rank, quoted in Choron, *Death and Modern Man*, p. 147.
32. Lois Jaffe, in *Dialogues*, p. 81.
33. Kapleau, editor, *Wheel of Death*, p. 67.
34. Max Weber, "Science as a Vocation," in H. H. Gerth and C. Wright Mills, editors, *From Max Weber*, pp. 139–40.
35. Siegel, *Love, Medicine & Miracles*, p. 208.
36. Grof and Halifax, *Human Encounter with Death*, p. 44.
37. Max Frisch, quoted in Karl Bloching, in Greinacher and Muller, editors, *Experience of Dying*, p. 29.
38. E. M. Forster, quoted in Lifton and Olson, *Living and Dying*, p. 37.
39. Diane Cole, *After Great Pain*, p. 131.
40. Hans Zinsser, *As I Remember Him*, p. 438.
41. Murray L. Trelease, in Kübler-Ross, editor, *Death*, p. 36.
42. Mwalimu Imara, in Kübler-Ross, editor, *Death*, pp. 152–53.

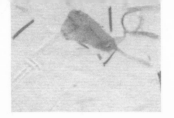

BIBLIOGRAPHY

Adler, Charles S., Gene Stanford, and Sheila Morrissey Adler, editors. *We Are But Moments of Sunlight: Understanding Death*. Pocket Books, New York, 1976.

Alsop, Stewart. *Stay of Execution: A Sort of Memoir*. Lippincott, Philadelphia, 1973.

Angier, Natalie. "The Transit of Woman," *New York Times Book Review,* October 11, 1992.

Ariès, Philippe. *The Hour of Our Death*. Knopf, New York, 1981.

———. *Western Attitudes Toward Death: From the Middle Ages to the Present*. Johns Hopkins University Press, Baltimore, 1974.

Beck, Melinda. "The New Middle Age," *Newsweek,* December 7, 1992.

Becker, Ernest. *The Denial of Death*. The Free Press, New York, 1973.

Beisser, Arnold R. *Flying Without Wings: Personal Reflections on Being Disabled*. Doubleday, New York, 1989.

Berman, Phillip L., editor. *The Courage to Grow Old*. Ballantine Books, New York, 1989.

Bluebond-Lagner, Myra. *The Private Worlds of Dying Children*. Princeton University Press, Princeton, N.J., 1978.

Boswell, James. *The Life of Samuel Johnson*. Doubleday, New York, 1946.

Brody, Howard. *Stories of Sickness*. Yale University Press, New Haven, Conn., 1987.

Brown, Norman O. *Life Against Death*. Vintage Books, New York, 1959.

Buchanan, James H. *Patient Encounters: The Experience of Disease*. University Press of Virginia, Charlottesville, 1988.

Choron, Jacques. *Death and Modern Man*. Collier Books, New York, 1964.

Clark, Etta. "Growing Old Is Not for Sissies," *The Sun,* Issue 196, March 1992.

Cole, Diane. *After Great Pain: A New Life Emerges.* Summit Books, New York, 1992.

Cousins, Norman. *Anatomy of an Illness as Perceived by the Patient.* Norton, New York, 1979.

————. *Head First: The Biology of Hope.* Dutton, New York, 1989.

————. *The Healing Heart: Antidotes to Panic and Helplessness.* Norton, New York, 1983.

Doernberg, Myrna. *Stolen Mind: The Slow Disappearance of Ray Doernberg.* Algonquin Books, Chapel Hill, N.C., 1986.

Erikson, Erik H., Joan M. Erikson, and Helen Q. Kivnik. *Vital Involvement in Old Age.* Norton, New York, 1986.

Feiden, Karyn. *Hope and Help for Chronic Fatigue Syndrome: The Official Guide of the CFS/CFIDS Network.* Prentice-Hall, New York, 1990.

Feifel, Herman, editor. *New Meanings of Death.* McGraw-Hill, New York, 1977.

Goshen-Gottstein, Esther. *Recalled to Life: The Story of a Coma.* Yale University Press, New Haven, Conn., 1990.

Greinacher, Norbert, and Alois Muller, editors. *The Experience of Dying.* Herder & Herder, New York, 1974.

Griffin, Moira. *Going the Distance: Living a Full Life with Multiple Sclerosis and Other Debilitating Diseases.* Dutton, New York, 1989.

Grof, Stanislav, and Joan Halifax. *The Human Encounter with Death.* Dutton, New York, 1977.

Hamilton, Clarence H., editor. *Buddhism: A Religion of Infinite Compassion.* Bobbs-Merrill, Indianapolis, 1952.

Heller, Joseph, and Speed Vogel. *No Laughing Matter.* Putnam, New York, 1986.

Howe, Herbert M. *Do Not Go Gentle.* Norton, New York, 1981.

Jury, Mark, and Dan Jury. *Gramp.* Grossman, New York, 1976.

Kalish, Richard A., editor. *Midlife Loss: Coping Strategies.* Sage, Newbury Park, Calif., 1989.

Kapleau, Philip, editor. *The Wheel of Death.* Harper & Row, New York, 1974.

Kavanaugh, Robert E. *Facing Death.* Nash, Los Angeles, 1972.

Kelly, Orville E. *Until Tomorrow Comes.* Everest House, New York, 1979.

Klawans, Harold L. *Toscanini's Fumble: And Other Tales of Clinical Neurology.* Contemporary Books, Chicago, 1988.

Kleinman, Arthur. *The Illness Narratives: Suffering, Healing and the Human Condition.* Basic Books, New York, 1988.

Koestler, Arthur, and John Raymond Smythies, editors. *Beyond Reductionism: New Perspectives in the Life Sciences.* Macmillan, New York, 1970.

Kotre, John, and Elizabeth Hall. *Seasons of Life.* Little, Brown, Boston, 1990.

Krementz, Jill. *How It Feels to Fight for Your Life.* Little, Brown, Boston, 1989.

Kübler-Ross, Elisabeth, editor. *Death: The Final Stage of Growth.* Prentice-Hall, Englewood Cliffs, N.J., 1975.

Kushner, Harold S. *When Bad Things Happen to Good People.* Schocken Books, New York, 1981.

Kutscher, Austin H., editor. *For the Bereaved: The Road to Recovery.* Princeton University Press, Princeton, N.J., 1990.

Kutscher, Austin H., Lillian G. Kutscher, et al., editors. *Dialogues: The Dying and the Living.* MSS Information Corp., Arno Press, New York, 1978.

Landon, H[oward] C[handler] Robbins, editor. *Beethoven: A Documentary Study.* Macmillan, New York, 1974.

Levitt, Paul M., and Elissa S. Guralnick. *You Can Make It Back: Coping with Serious Illness.* Facts on File, New York, 1985.

Lifton, Robert Jay, and Eric Olson. *Living and Dying.* Praeger, New York, 1974.

McLeish, John A. B. *The Ulyssean Adult: Creativity in the Middle and Later Years.* McGraw-Hill Ryerson, Ltd., Toronto, 1976.

Marks, Elaine. *Simone de Beauvoir: Encounters with Death.* Rutgers University Press, New Brunswick, N.J., 1973.

Marris, Peter. *Loss and Change.* Anchor Books, Garden City, N.Y., 1975.

Maurer, Janet, and Patricia D. Strasberg. *Building a New Dream: A Family Guide to Coping with Chronic Illness and Disability.* Addison-Wesley, Reading, Mass., 1989.

Montaigne, Michel Eyquem de. *The Essays.* Encyclopaedia Britannica, Chicago, 1952.

Newsweek. "Menopause," May 25, 1992.

Newsweek. "The Young and the Restless," January 11, 1993.

Petrow, Steven. *Dancing Against the Darkness: A Journey Through America in the Age of AIDS.* Lexington Books, Lexington, Mass., 1990.

Pitts, Beverly J., and Mark N. Popovich. "Aftermath of an NFL Career: Injuries." Unpublished manuscript.

Pitts, Beverly, Mark N. Popovich, and Anthony T. Bober. "Life After Football: A Survey of Former NFL Players." Unpublished manuscript, May 1989.

Pressley, Nelson. "His Cheatin' Art," *Washington Post,* August 23, 1992.

Raphael, Beverly. *The Anatomy of Bereavement.* Basic Books, New York, 1983.

Rollin, Betty. *First, You Cry.* Lippincott, Philadelphia, 1976.

——. *Last Wish.* Linden Press, New York, 1985.

Rosenfeld, Stephen S. *The Time of Their Dying.* Norton, New York, 1977.

Rush, John. *Beating Depression.* Facts on File, New York, 1983.

Sacks, Oliver. *The Man Who Mistook His Wife for a Hat.* Summit Books, New York, 1985.

Shapiro, Kenneth A. *Dying and Living.* University of Texas Press, Austin, 1985.

Sherman, Edmund. *Meaning in Mid-Life Transitions.* State University of New York Press, Albany, 1987.

Shneidman, Edwin S., editor. *Death: Current Perspectives.* Mayfield, Palo Alto, Calif., 1984.

——. *Deaths of Man.* Quadrangle, New York, 1973.

Siegel, Bernie S. *Love, Medicine & Miracles: Lessons Learned About Self-Healing from a Surgeon's Experience with Exceptional Patients.* Harper & Row, New York, 1986.

Sourkes, Barbara M. *The Deepening Shade: Psychological Aspects of Life-Threatening Illness.* University of Pittsburgh Press, Pittsburgh, 1982.

Styron, William. *Darkness Visible: A Memoir of Madness.* Random House, New York, 1990.

Stryk, Lucien, comp. *World of the Buddha: A Reader.* Doubleday/Anchor, New York, 1969.

Szasz, Suzy. *Living with It: Why You Don't Have to Be Healthy to Be Happy.* Prometheus Books, Buffalo, N.Y., 1991.

Tatelbaum, Judy. *The Courage to Grieve.* Lippincott & Crowell, New York, 1980.

Taylor, Charles, editor. *Growing On: Ideas About Aging.* Van Nostrand Reinhold, New York, 1984.

Tournier, Paul. *Learn to Grow Old.* Harper & Row, New York, 1972.

Viorst, Judith. *Necessary Losses.* Simon & Schuster, New York, 1986.

Weber, Max. "Science as a Vocation," in Gerth, H. H., and C. Wright Mills, editors. *From Max Weber: Essays in Sociology.* Routledge and Kegan Paul, London, 1948.

Woolf, Virginia. *The Moment and Other Essays.* Harcourt Brace, New York, 1948.

Zinsser, Hans. *As I Remember Him: The Biography of R. S.* Little, Brown, Boston, 1940.

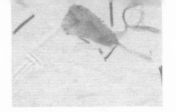

INDEX